Down Syndrome

Down Syndrome
Moving through life

Edited by
Yvonne Burns

Physiotherapy Department
University of Queensland
Brisbane, Australia

and

Pat Gunn

Fred and Eleanor Schonell Special Education Research Centre
University of Queensland
Brisbane, Australia

CHAPMAN & HALL
London · Glasgow · New York · Tokyo · Melbourne · Madras

Published by Chapman & Hall, 2–6 Boundary Row, London SE1 8HN

Chapman & Hall, 2–6 Boundary Row, London SE1 8HN, UK

Blackie Academic & Professional, Wester Cleddens Road, Bishopbriggs, Glasgow G64 2NZ, UK

Chapman & Hall Inc., 29 West 35th Street, New York NY10001, USA

Chapman & Hall Japan, Thomson Publishing Japan, Hirakawacho Nemoto Building, 6F, 1–7–11 Hirakawa-cho, Chiyoda-ku, Tokyo 102, Japan

Chapman & Hall Australia, Thomas Nelson Australia, 102 Dodds Street, South Melbourne, Victoria 3205, Australia

Chapman & Hall India, R. Seshadri, 32 Second Main Road, CIT East, Madras 600 035, India

Distributed in the USA and Canada by Singular Publishing Group Inc., 4284 41st Street, San Diego, California 92105, USA

First edition 1993

© 1993 Chapman & Hall

Typeset in 10/12 pt Palatino by Mews Photosetting, Beckenham, Kent
Printed in Great Britain by St Edmundsbury Press,
Bury St Edmunds, Suffolk

ISBN 0 412 46180 3   1 56593 140 8 (USA)

A catalogue record for this book is available from the British Library

Library of Congress Cataloging-in-Publication data

Down syndrome : moving through life / edited by Yvonne Burns and
    Pat Gunn. – 1st ed.
        p. cm.
    Includes bibliographical references and indexes.
    ISBN 0-412-46180-3 (acid-free paper)
    Down syndrome – Patients – Rehabilitation. 2. Physical
education for mentally handicapped persons. 3. Movement education.
I. Burns, Yvonne. II. Gunn, Pat.
RC571.D686 1993
616.85′8842–dc20   **173715**   93-18675
                                                         CIP

∞ Printed on permanent acid-free text paper, manufactured in accordance with the proposed ANSI/NISO Z 39.48-199X and ANSI Z 39.48-1984

Contents

Contributors

Sue Price
Yeronga Physiotherapy
Yeronga Village
12 Kadumba Street
Yeronga 4104
Australia

Rose-Anne Kelso
Yeronga Physiotherapy
Yeronga Village
12 Kadumba Street
Yeronga 4104
Australia

Louise Mercer
Physiotherapist
Low Incidence Support Centre
72 Cornwall Street
Annerley 4103
Australia

Anne Jobling
Fred and Eleanor Schonell Special Education
    Research Centre
The University of Queensland
Brisbane 4072
Australia

Dr Jenny Ziviani
Occupational Therapy Department
The University of Queensland
Brisbane 4072
Australia

Prof. John Elkins
Fred and Eleanor Schonell Special Education
    Research Centre
The University of Queensland
Brisbane 4072
Australia

Pamela Barham
Network Coaching International
7 Maher Street
Sunshine Beach 4567
Australia

Dr Barbara James
Division of Workplace Health and Safety
50 Ann Street
Brisbane 4000
Australia

Preface

The intent of this book is to suggest activities that will foster the development of efficient and effective patterns of movement in persons with Down syndrome. Attention to the nature of movement patterns is especially important for those with Down syndrome as their motor milestones are usually delayed and patterns of movement vary in quality. The book outlines principles and practices that have gained from co-operation between therapists, teachers, and other professionals. All chapters have been written by a professional in the relevant discipline who has had extensive experience with Down syndrome.

We believe that the book would be suitable as a supplementary text for final year undergraduate and postgraduate students and of interest to professionals concerned with movement including physiotherapists, occupational therapists, and physical education teachers. We hope that parents and friends of persons with Down syndrome will find the chapters useful and informative.

The chapters have taken a global perspective, not only by considering movement through the lifespan but movement for function, for school learning, for work, leisure and recreation. Many of the suggestions will be appropriate for other forms of developmental disability, especially those with hypotonia and developmental delay.

The overall theme of the book reflects the belief that an interdisciplinary focus on the quality of movement and the development of motor skills in persons with Down syndrome will make a major contribution towards their personal competence and increased participation in the activities of the wider community.

Yvonne Burns
Pat Gunn

Acknowledgements

We thank the parents, children and adults who consented to be photographed. Their contribution to the chapters is very much appreciated and there is no doubt that their photos have enlivened the printed words. We are further indebted to many others with Down syndrome who do not appear in the photos but who have had a marked influence on us, our assumptions and our values, and whose aspirations underpin the purpose of this book.

For permission to reprint photographs, we thank the Fred and Eleanor Schonell Special Education Research Centre, University of Queensland, for the photographs in Chapters three and four; the Courier Mail, Brisbane, Queensland for photograph 6.3 in Chapter six; Project Recreation, Ipswich, Queensland for photographs 8.4 and 8.5 in Chapter eight and 9.2 in Chapter nine; Ausrapid, Victoria for photograph 9.1 in Chapter nine.

Finally, P.G. thanks her husband for his tolerant understanding of editorial preoccupations and his insistence on plain English.

1

Characteristics of Down syndrome

Pat Gunn

INTRODUCTION

Down syndrome occurs in all parts of the world. It is not restricted to any one race, culture, social class, or historical period. Evidence of the syndrome dates back to artefacts of the Olmecs in ancient Mexico (Stratford, 1989) although the first detailed and systematic description by Langdon Down came much later, in 1866.

Almost 100 years after this description, Lejeune *et al.* (1959) counted 47 chromosomes in the cells of nine children. This important discovery stimulated dramatic changes in knowledge about the syndrome and led to positive diagnosis by karyotype analysis. Until then, the diagnosis had been based on the constellation of physical features reported by Down. Yet, although there are several physical signs associated with the syndrome there are none which exactly define it. Indeed, only a few years before Lejeune *et al.*'s report, Øster (1953) had written that it was impossible to define the condition as 'opinion is divided as to which features and how many ought to be included' (p. 15).

The 47 chromosomes found by Lejeune *et al.* arose from the presence of an extra chromosome 21, a result of meiotic non-disjunction. More recent improvements in cytogenetic techniques have shown that this non-disjunction is sometimes of paternal origin (Abroms and Bennett, 1981) and that the region of the chromosome linked to Down syndrome is the distal segment 21q22. Other findings include a genetic link between chromosome 21 and certain conditions such as cataracts, leukaemia, and Alzheimer's disease (Groner *et al.*, 1986; Patterson, 1987). Current research is directed towards further mapping of the genes on chromosome 21 as a preliminary step towards understanding the effects of the extra genetic material.

Along with this growth in knowledge about the nature of the syndrome, there have been noteworthy changes in the life prospects of people with Down syndrome. In many countries, children with Down syndrome are now reared at home instead of facing life in institutions or hospitals while adults are being encouraged to greater independence within their own communities. Moreover, advances in medical treatment have overcome many health problems and reports around the world have indicated longer and healthier lives (Masaki *et al.*, 1981; Thase, 1982a; Stratford and Steele, 1985; Fryers, 1986; Dupont *et al.*, 1986; Malone, 1988; Eyman *et al.*, 1991).

During this increased life span, the person with Down syndrome will be seen as a member of the everyday community rather than as a resident of a special facility. The adolescent with Down syndrome will make the transition from school to employment or further education and will participate in community activities through adult life. Whether this life is allied to social acceptance and personal satisfaction will depend to some extent on the degree to which the person is successful in meeting everyday challenges at home and in the community. These challenges may be in the form of employment, self care or recreational activities but the common basis for a successful outcome is competent motor behaviour. The basic actions of posture, locomotion, and manipulation are involved in tasks which range from assembly work, gardening, playing the piano or playing netball, to writing a message or eating with a knife and fork.

Incompetent motor behaviour not only hinders the person's ability to succeed with everyday activities but can have a negative impact on personal satisfaction and social acceptance. Personal satisfaction is related to successful achievement but the self confidence of many young people is also influenced by their own appearance and their comparison with various role models, often TV stars. Obesity, awkward gait, clumsiness, fine motor skills too poor for legible handwriting or useful handiwork, and bizarre movement patterns are unlikely to contribute to successful achievement, social acceptance, or personal satisfaction.

If such maladaptive attributes are to be avoided, effective and efficient patterns of movement need to be established during childhood. The enhancement of the quality of movement and the motor competence of the child with Down syndrome is related not only to ongoing childhood activities but also to later development as an adult. The avoidance of aberrant or detrimental habits of movement and the development of useful motor skills can make a positive contribution to the well-being of the older individual and lead to enhanced participation in community life. This is a general statement which can be applied to everyone, not only to those with Down syndrome.

Indeed it is important to recognize that the main attribute which distinguishes people with Down syndrome from everyone else is the additional complement of chromosome 21 genes. It may also be added that all people with Down syndrome are not identical, even with respect to this extra genetic material. The majority have a total of 47 chromosomes because of an additional chromosome 21 (trisomy 21). A few people have an extra 21q22 segment attached to another chromosome (translocation). Mosaicism is a third, but even less common form of Down syndrome, in which some cells have the normal complement of 46 chromosomes but because of errors in later cell division, other cells show trisomy 21.

The path of development for each individual depends not only on the effects of the extra genetic material but also on the mediating influence of other genetic material and environmental factors. Physical appearance reflects family likeness, not only syndrome 'signs'. Cognitive level varies from that typical of severe intellectual disability to almost average competence. Personalities include the pleasant and easy-going as well as the difficult and unpredictable. Interests vary with age and experience. Skills depend on opportunities and practice.

Most of the early literature tended to portray the characteristics in syndrome specific terms and there was little acknowledgement of these individual differences. There is now a better understanding that, although syndrome specific characteristics may be delineated (Gibson, 1989, 1991), the variability in individual development must be acknowledged (Barden 1983; Crombie *et al.*, 1991; Hayes and Gunn, 1991).

As far as motor competence is concerned, this variability is mirrored in the ages reported for motor milestones. For example, the range given for sitting without support is from six to 16 months and for walking alone is from 13 to more than 48 months (Cunningham, 1982). It is not only with respect to the age at which such motor milestones are attained that there are wide individual differences but there seem also to be individual differences regarding the physical or perceptual deficits which may subvert the skill. As Henderson (1987) concluded, 'What we can do positively is reject the notion that a single deficit might underlie all the behaviour manifestations of motor delay and incompetence which we observe in Down's individuals.' (p. 213). Henderson also pointed out that explanations for these various manifestations could not be tested until we had an adequate theory of motor development.

SYSTEMS APPROACHES TO MOVEMENT

More recently, there has been a resurgence of interest in theories of motor development. In a special issue of *Developmental Psychology*, von Hofsten (1989) summarized two main approaches. The first, the perception-action systems approach, is based on a close link between perception and goal directed actions. Reed (1989) provides an example. 'What enables a normal person to be able to use a fork standing, seated, lying down, with different-sized bites, and so on, is the ability to use available perceptual information to adapt both posture and movement allowing use of a fork in any given instance.' (p. 21).

The second approach described by von Hofsten, the dynamic systems approach, is more concerned with morphological questions and explanations for transitions in development. For example, as Thelen and Ulrich (1991) observed 'the motivational aspect of locomoting towards a desired goal is independent of the means of achieving that goal. Infants will scoot, roll, shuffle, creep, crawl or use a wheeled device to reach a desired object often six months or more before they walk. It is not the translation of intention into motor action that limits locomotion but the developmental readiness of the sensory and neuromotor elements needed for particular postures and actions.' (pp. 40–41).

Both the perception-action systems approach and the dynamic systems approach regard movement as an expression of the interaction of multiple subsystems. Thelen (1989) has argued that this emphasis is not surprising given that 'For a child to move, perception, motivation, plans, physiological status and affect must all interact with a mechanical system that is composed of muscles, bones and joints. Although we may not choose to study all these contributing elements at the same time, it is conceptually impossible (and empirically foolish) to encapsulate the movement outcome from the motives that inspired it, the information that guided it, and the body parts that produced it.' (p. 946).

The necessity of considering all these contributing elements has important implications for those who initiate activity programmes with children or adults with Down syndrome.

Information guiding the movement

'Making successful movements involves knowledge of the world and of one's position within it, so it is not possible to understand movement and action if perception is not considered too.' (Smyth, 1984, p. 119).

A variety of studies related to the visual perception of infants and young children with Down syndrome have been reported. Some have indicated that infants with Down syndrome seem to prefer patterns of low complexity (Miranda and Fantz, 1973; 1974) and have problems in switching visual attention (Gunn *et al.*, 1982; Krakow and Kopp, 1982; Kasari *et al.*, 1990). Landry and Chapieski (1990) reported that it was easier to elicit their attention than to redirect it.

At 12 months of age, these children show less manual exploration than other children (Vietze *et al.*, 1983) and at school age they have difficulty with tasks which demand attention to more than one dimension, e.g. size and pattern (Stratford, 1987).

Anwar (1981) has suggested that children with Down syndrome are efficient in using proprioceptive feedback and that strategies adopted during training through the kinaesthetic/

proprioceptive system may transfer to the visual system. Henderson (1987), however, emphasized the way in which Anwar had systematically guided the child's finger around each stimulus. She suggested that this guidance helped to draw the child's attention to the shape and that this, rather than an efficient proprioceptive system, had improved the child's ability to process the shape information. 'Therefore, when the child's attention was drawn to that source of information and organized for him, it became manageable.' (p. 201).

Although studies of visual perception have ranged from laboratory measures of infant visual preferences to observations of the direction of child looking in free play situations and tests of recognition which involve visual or proprioceptive information, one overall conclusion seems to be that children with Down syndrome are inefficient regarding their attention strategies. They seem not to benefit from incidental learning and may need help in directing attention to the relevant cues. They may have particular difficulty with complex relationships when more than one dimension or more than one modality is to be processed.

Another series of studies has been concerned with the integration of vision with postural control. Butterworth and his colleagues (Butterworth and Hicks, 1977; Butterworth and Cicchetti, 1978) explored the relationship between visual feedback and postural stability in infants with Down syndrome who had just learned either to sit or to stand and Shumway-Cook and Woollacott (1985) extended the study to older children. The results indicated that children with Down syndrome had difficulty in compensating for perceptual discrepancies. Their postural control responses were slower and the older standing children swayed more and fell over more than other children in response to conflicting sensory inputs. Another study related to these findings has been conducted by Rast and Harris (1985) who reported that the emergence of postural righting reactions was delayed and that the movements for head control were different for infants with Down syndrome.

In explaining their results, Butterworth and Cicchetti suggested that the vestibular system of infants with Down syndrome may require a high level of stimulation before it can detect discrepancies between mechanical-vestibular and visual sources of information. They also observed that failures in early postural control will impede the development of later postures and that a deficit in the postural control system leads to motor problems in everyday functioning. For example, the development of fine motor skills will be hampered by the delay in gaining control of the trunk while sitting.

Other studies of perceptual functioning in Down syndrome have been concerned with auditory processing. Measurements of event-related potentials to auditory stimuli led Lincoln *et al.* (1985) to the conclusion that 'children with Down syndrome have significant impairment in (a) the speed of orienting to and categorizing auditory information, (b) the organization of a motor response, and (c) the processes necessary for utilizing immediate auditory memory' (p. 413).

The results of a study using different techniques led Varnhagen *et al.* (1987) to the conclusion that the deficit in auditory processing in adults with Down syndrome may be traced to a delay in accessing information in long-term memory and to difficulties in storing phonological information.

A related area of research stems from studies of dichotic listening and is concerned with the possibility that there is a unique pattern of cerebral specialization in Down syndrome (Hartley, 1986). Other studies have suggested that there may be special difficulties with tasks which require both perception of speech and production of movement (Elliott *et al.*, 1987; Elliott, 1990).

One practical implication of these studies of auditory processing appears to be that a person with Down syndrome will benefit from being given extra time to process verbal instructions and from being given a limited amount of information to process in any one instruction, especially if it requires a motor response. A demonstration may add further clarity to short, concise instructions.

Timing seems to have special implications for the motor competency of those with Down syndrome. Henderson (1987) concluded that people with Down syndrome are slow and lack precision on timed tasks. She suggested that they have special difficulty in altering the pace of movement and in producing fast movements. According to Henderson, this is not due solely to cognitive decision factors but there are delays at the neuromotor level as well. These timing difficulties have most effect on proficiency in changing or unstable situations. Such situations include games in which there is a need not only to run fast or throw accurately but also to dodge an opponent or throw to a moving partner (Sugden and Keogh, 1990). They also include employment tasks which demand speed and variety of execution rather than thoroughness and repetition.

Motivation and affect

Although the previous studies have been concerned with perceptual processing and motor planning, some of the findings integrate well with the literature on motivation and temperament. Reports in this literature of reduced task persistence, depressed arousal/activation thresholds, motivation difficult to sustain, and error perseveration are not difficult to reconcile with attentional deficits, auditory processing deficits, and difficulties with timed tasks and motor precision.

The evidence for reduced task persistence comes from a variety of studies. It includes temperament ratings that reflect low persistence in infants as well as in adolescents (Gunn and Berry, 1985; Gunn and Cuskelly, 1991), low persistence by infants on tasks near the limits of their competence (Schwethelm and Mahoney, 1986), and in comparison with other infants, less time spent on task mastery (MacTurk *et al.*, 1985).

Duffy and Wishart (1987) discussed the motivational characteristics of children with Down syndrome, six to ten years of age, who took part in a study in which different strategies were used to teach discrimination skills. In comparison with others, the children with Down syndrome learnt best by errorless training but they consistently showed evidence of switching out of cognitive tasks. Duffy and Wishart suggested motivational factors to explain their results and described the poor performance of the older children as a case of 'won't do' rather than 'can't do'. Recently, Wishart (1991) has reported similar avoidance behaviours in a study with infants six to 24 months of age.

Fear or failure and lower expectancies of success have been interpreted as causes of low persistence in older children and adults with intellectual disabilities but it is difficult to reconcile this explanation with the reduced task persistence shown by infants with Down syndrome. At first sight, these children would seem to be too young for their past experiences to provide a satisfactory explanation in terms of previous failure. On the other hand, in these days of early intervention, many infants with Down syndrome are presented with tasks to be mastered almost from the day they are born. These experiences may not be associated with failure, but the artificially high rates of encouragement which accompany these tasks may make it difficult for the child to determine a link between praise and effort. At all ages, it is important to link praise appropriately to the effort rather than to give indiscriminate social reinforcement.

Wishart found that her assessments with the Bayley Scales of Infant Development were affected by the irregular performance of children with Down syndrome. It is interesting to consider her results in terms of the social meaning to the child following the example of Hogg (1986) who used von Cranach's (1982) model of cognition, behaviour, and social meaning to discuss the results of a preschool study by Moss and Hogg (1983). These authors found greater variety in manipulation sequences with the growth of child competence and contrasted this finding with observations by Dalgleish (1977) of decreasing variety in strategies as the child became more proficient in spoon use.

Hogg suggested that the variety in the Moss and Hogg study may have arisen because the children had interpreted the social meaning of their manipulation tasks as 'play' in contrast to the functional meaning of spoon use. This is an important suggestion and the child's perception of the assessment or therapy task and its contingencies may well have more explanatory value for child behaviour than is usually conceded.

Mundy *et al.* (1988) have further suggested that low arousal and a passive style of behaviour contribute to deficits in the motivation of children with Down syndrome while Gibson and Fields (1984) have argued that low reactivity invited low stimulation resulting in 'progressive abatement of development' (p. 358).

A variety of studies have found that babies with Down syndrome are slow in responding to smiling or laughter (Cicchetti and Sroufe, 1976; Sorce and Emde, 1982) and this literature suggests that stimulation may need to be more intrusive than usual to compensate for the infant's passivity. The ease with which interactions become a source of mutual enjoyment has been acknowledged as a source of maternal satisfaction. It seems reasonable also to assume that it is the enjoyable interchanges which will motivate the child for further interaction.

An interesting relationship between hypotonia and laughter has been reported by Cicchetti and Sroufe (1976) who found that babies with marked hypotonia showed least smiling and the onset of their laughter was much later than that for other infants with Down syndrome. These children responded to intense physical activity rather than to more subtle forms of playful stimulation.

The physical system

There are some important features of the physical system that are distinctive for Down syndrome and which impinge on the development of motor competence. Children with Down syndrome are well below average in height for their age group although most of the height deficit occurs before puberty. Rapid changes in height at puberty occur at much the same age as other children and the rate of change at that time is just below that for their peers. Their short stature is reported to be a reflection of short leg length rather than short sitting height (Rarick and Seefeldt, 1974). Not only are the long bones of the leg shorter than the norm, so too are those in the arms and digits. These body proportions need to be considered for their possible effects on strength, posture, locomotion and manipulation.

Other features include the persistence of primitive reflexes and generalized muscular hypotonia. Cowie (1970) clinically assessed muscle tone by the resistance to passive stretch of the limbs, palpation of the muscle mass, various postures, and flexibility. She found every infant in her sample hypotonic and attributed later deficits in motor skills to the underlying hypotonia.

Shumway-Cook and Woollacott (1985) have queried this assumption as their study of tonic activity and myotatic reflexes during platform displacement suggested that postural control problems in children with Down syndrome did not result from hypotonia. Their results were consistent with those of Davis and his colleagues who found muscle stiffness in Down syndrome, though not as easily activated, was comparable to normal development (Davis and Kelso, 1982; Davis and Sinning, 1987). Davis and Kelso concluded that the nature of the association between muscle tone and motor performance deficiencies was obscure. They noted, however, the inconsistency of measuring tone during passive movement while trying to determine its effect on active performance.

Although both hypotonia and excessive joint flexibility are reported consistently in infants with Down syndrome, many writers have reported improvements with age (Morris *et al.*, 1982; Harris, 1984; Parker and James, 1985).

Another important aspect of the physical system concerns the nature of the health problems associated with Down syndrome. The most serious of these are congenital heart defects which have been reported in about one third of the children born with Down syndrome. Until recently, these were the major determinant of survival but advances in medical care and surgical treatment have improved this outlook considerably (Malone, 1988).

Nevertheless, Reed *et al.* (1980) reported that children with congenital heart disease were less active and more lethargic than other children with Down syndrome. They suggested three possible reasons for the depressed activity levels, the cardiac work load, medications which reduce appetite hence available energy, and the common fear of parents that activity may harm the child.

There is no doubt that a cardiological check-up and modification of vigorous activities have to be considered in some cases. This does not imply, however, that active participation in games or exercises should be avoided. In Hallidie-Smith's (1987) view, 'only very rarely is exercise dangerous for a child with a heart defect, and, if such a situation exists, as in severe aortic stenosis, the treatment is surgical relief.' (pp. 66–67). She suggested that children learn their own limits and so restrict the activities themselves.

A number of orthopaedic problems which impact on motor competence have been reported. Instability at the atlanto-axial joint, however, is potentially the most severe of these problems as it can lead to dislocation of the vertebrae with the atlas sliding forward over the axis. This can lead to damage of the spinal cord due to compression by the odontoid process of the axis. Reports have indicated that instability occurs in 9–22% of children and adults with Down syndrome and about 2% may sustain neurological damage to the spinal cord (Tredwell *et al.*, 1990). Symptoms of such damage may include abnormal neurological findings such as a positive Babinski reflex, ankle clonus, abnormal gait, inability to walk, rigid or tilted head, and progressive quadriparesis (Howard, 1985).

Alvarez and Rubin (1986) advocated routine screening of patients with Down syndrome as the potentially crippling, and possibly fatal complication of spinal cord compression can be prevented by early detection and prompt management.' (p. 74).

The atlanto-axial instability has been attributed mainly to laxity of the transverse ligaments and is usually determined radiographically by measuring the distance between the atlas and the odontoid process of the axis in hyperflexion. Those who have a gap of 5 mm or more but who do not show compression symptoms are regarded as asymptomatic. It is advisable for this group to be examined regularly for signs of neurological damage and to have annual neck X-rays (Selikowitz, 1990). It is also advisable to avoid activities such as diving, butterfly stroke when swimming, gymnastics (tumbling), high jump, pentathlon, soccer and any exercise which places pressure on the neck or head muscles (Committee on Sports Medicine, 1984).

For those few who do show symptoms of spinal cord compression, surgery has been recommended to fuse the back of the atlas to the back of the axis. This reduces the mobility of the neck but need not lead to a sedentary life.

Because of the tendency to poor muscle tone and ligament laxity, degenerative changes are likely to be found in the joints, especially those that are weight bearing. Some evidence of this conclusion has been provided by Diamond *et al.* (1981) who found forefoot abnormalities, scoliosis, disclocation of the patella, and dislocation of the hips among the orthopaedic problems of adults with Down syndrome. Degenerative changes in the spine of older adults also have been reported by Jagjivan *et al.* (1988).

Several writers have considered the tendency for children and adults with Down syndrome to be overweight. Some have suggested that the stature of the person with Down syndrome may contribute to the appearance of obesity because of the short leg length/stature ratio. Others have investigated the caloric intake (Chad *et al.*, 1990) and the basal metabolic rate (Schapiro and Rapoport, 1989). It seems that the basal metabolic rate is not affected in trisomy 21 and that inactivity rather than excessive food intake may be the main reason for obesity. Pueschel (1988) has warned of the vicious circle between weight gain, avoidance of activity, more sedentary pursuits, more snacking and further weight gain. He has cautioned that obesity has both health related and non-health related concerns. The former concerns include a higher frequency of diabetes, increased blood pressure, and a reduced life expectancy. The latter concerns encompass reduced participation in social and recreational experiences and increased social stigma.

It is important to make the distinction between obesity and hypothyroidism and between Down syndrome and hypothyroidism. The thyroid has an overall effect on level of activity or sluggishness and hypothyroidism has a permanent deleterious effect on intellectual functioning. Many countries test thyroid hormone levels at birth or soon after and it has been recommended that this be repeated annually for everyone with Down syndrome, as hypothyroidism is found frequently in infants and children with Down syndrome and even more often in adults (Fort *et al.*, 1984; Pueschel and Pezzullo, 1985; Selikowitz, 1990).

Sensory deficits have been reported for Down syndrome and these will require treatment if optimal development is to be attained. Hearing loss has been found in children (Dahle and McCollister, 1986), in adults (Keiser *et al.* 1981), and in children and adults with Down syndrome (Brooks *et al.*, 1972; Balkany *et al.* 1979). The incidence of impairment in these studies has varied from 15 to 50% so that a high proportion of those with Down syndrome are likely to have experienced the negative effects of hearing impairment on communication and interpersonal relationships (Libb *et al.*, 1985; Whiteman *et al.*, 1986).

The hearing loss is most often due to conductive impairment and has been attributed to a high incidence of recurrent otitis media with fluid accumulation in the middle ear. The aetiology lies in eustachian tube dysfunction which is associated with anatomic abnormalities of the eustachian tube and its surrounding facial structures (Giebink and Daly, 1990). Keiser *et al.* found that most adults in their sample had mixed conductive and sensorineural loss. Brooks *et al.* found an association between age and type of loss. They conjectured that sensorineural loss was due to long standing middle ear problems and perhaps preventable if diagnosed early. Out of 38 patients with Down syndrome less than 20 years of age, only 21% had sensorineural loss whereas among 40 patients more than 21 years of age, 55% had sensorineural loss (Wisniewski *et al.*, 1988).

Other sensory impairments include those related to vision. Pueschel (1987) reported incidence figures for congenital cataracts (3%), refractive errors (77%), strabismus (49%), nystagmus (35%) and blocked tear duct (20%). The importance of monitoring and correcting impairments in hearing and vision has been indicated by Hewitt and Jancar (1986) who found that decreased visual acuity and hearing loss were strongly associated with intellectual decline in a group of 23 patients with Down syndrome aged over 50 years.

Alzheimer morphology has been commonly reported in older persons with Down syndrome but it is not possible to conclude that all develop Alzheimer's Disease. Schweber (1987) reported that up to three-fourths of those with Down syndrome who showed signs of Alzheimer's at autopsy had not developed significant mental problems with age. It seems that a distinction should be made between neuropathological and clinical signs of Alzheimer's and, 'it should never be assumed that Alzheimer's disease is the invariant consequence of longevity in Down syndrome.' (p. 361, Thase, 1988). Sensory impairment e.g. cataracts or hearing loss may produce cognitive or behavioural changes in the older adult (Hewitt *et al.*, 1985) and thyroid imbalance, other illnesses, depression, and medication should be investigated regarding their possible influence on behaviour (Thase, 1982b).

LEARNING

The previous paragraphs have been concerned with the

characteristics of Down syndrome which may influence motor performance. The question as to how those with Down syndrome can be helped to acquire proficiency or skill in performance also needs to be addressed. Henderson (1987) pointed out, however, that there has been a tendency for the focus of research into Down syndrome motor development to be on performance rather than on learning.

Recent theories of skill acquisition have emphasized self-generated exploration by the learner rather than the reproduction of a stereotyped action. Through this exploration, the learner develops the ability to use perceptual information from a variety of contexts and to co-ordinate this information with the movements and posture needed to meet task requirements. An example is Connolly and Dalgleish's (1989) detailed description of children learning to use a spoon. The children found many different initial solutions to the problem but what was stable was the goal and the functionally rewarding practice. In designing therapy and physical education programmes, it is not just a matter of applying task analysis to the skill to be taught and then teaching each component in sequence but the learner's self-generated strategies and the goal with its functional rewards should be considered also.

It has been proposed by Newell (1991) that there are three components to be considered in understanding the acquisition of skill. One concerns the self-generated or natural exploration strategies of the learner (akin to discovery learning as in solving the problem of using a spoon efficiently). The second concerns the nature of the perceptual-motor workspace, the co-ordination of perceptual information with an understanding of the movements required for the task and the third concerns the use of augmented information to facilitate the learner's exploration.

In the case of the learner with Down syndrome, the most effective augmentation will consider the information processing, arousal, motivational, and physical characteristics that are specific to the syndrome (Gibson, 1991). The nature of the augmented information will also depend on the stage of learning, for example postural support for young infants will enhance visual exploration and reaching but more advanced learners will require different forms of support for more complex tasks.

One common form of augmented information is the physical guidance provided by a therapist or teacher who moves a child through the actions to be learned. Such a procedure will be counter-productive if the child resists and the need to be aware of the learner's perceptions of the procedures should be paramount. The goal is towards self-directed activity and this is unlikely to be achieved if the teaching or therapy procedures are aversive.

The more advanced learner may not need manual guidance but will benefit from demonstration or from verbal instructions. In this case it is necessary to bear in mind that a person with Down syndrome may have a hearing loss or an auditory processing difficulty. Instructions should be short and for those who have most difficulty in acquiring aural/oral language skills, sign language may be used for communication. If visual cues are used to augment information, it would be advisable to reduce their complexity so that attention is not required for multiple dimensions.

The relationship of the functional reward to the acquisition of skill seems to have been recognized particularly in the literature on severe intellectual disabilities. Sailor *et al.* (1988) have argued that context relevance is a source of motivation which leads to generalization and maintenance of the newly learned skills of students with severe disabilities. As the basis for context relevance, these authors have suggested that the skill to be learned has to be useful, desirable, practical and appropriate for the student. The skill should also be acquired in a social context and in the physical contexts in which it will ultimately be requested. These authors provided an example of a mobility skill which was learned by four students with severe disabilities within actual travel routes rather than through training prerequisite skills in a sequence. The functional value of the goal seems to have underpinned this achievement as it did for younger children as they improved their skill with a spoon.

Practice is fundamental to the maintenance of a newly learned skill and is especially important for those with intellectual disabilities. Kerr and Blais (1988) have demonstrated that aspects of the motor performance of young adults with Down syndrome can be maximized with extended practice. In their study, the practice was structured by a teacher but spontaneous practice by the learner would appear to have even more desirable benefits for maintenance and for generalization. If spontaneous practice is to be encouraged, its value to the learner must be considered. There may be times when this lies in the functional value of the goal (as in the previous examples) and other times when it lies in the enjoyment of the activity.

Hogg (1981) found that preschool children during their free play showed little spontaneous use of the skills they had learnt in a structured teaching situation and concluded that the motor activities which the child enjoyed should determine the tasks in a motor development curriculum. These ideas have been expanded by Vallerand and Reid (1990) who considered ways in which spontaneous physical activity can be encouraged even if the person's initial interest in the activity is not high. These authors stressed the necessity of promoting the learner's feelings of competence and discussed the provision of choices, goal setting, co-operative games, and peer modelling as possible motivational devices.

Although there is still much to be learned about skill development in children and adults with Down syndrome, it would appear that effective guidance overcomes passivity and encourages children and adults to take a more active role in their own learning. The value of the procedures to the child or adult must never be forgotten in the therapy and teaching programmes. The motivation to achieve a set task will depend on the perspective of the learner and not on the perspective of the therapist, teacher, or caregiver. It must also be emhasized that every person with Down syndrome is an individual and that the most effective therapy or teaching programme will capitalize on this individuality.

2

The development of movement: the basis of effective performance and life skills

Yvonne Burns

INTRODUCTION

The first five years in the life of a child is a period of spectacular change in growth and development. Although within the first days and weeks following birth the young infant can respond to touch, sound, taste, handling and visual images especially the human face, the baby is totally dependent on a carer for protection, nourishment, support against gravity, and movement throughout the environment. Within a few years, however, most children are totally physically independent, able to control their balance, perform a wide variety of gross and fine motor activities and learn new skills requiring a high degree of control and perception.

All aspects of the remarkable development of function are inter-related but for the purpose of clarity this chapter will concentrate on those aspects which specifically relate to the development of posture, movement and motor control. Throughout this discussion reference will be made to some typical problems experienced by infants and children with Down syndrome. It is important however, to realize that many children with Down syndrome will display none or only some of these difficulties or differences while others may experience additional problems. A later section on assessment will address the recognition or identification of specific movement problems. Guidelines and philosophies of intervention aimed at enhancing an individual's potential abilities and functional independence will be presented.

The process of motor development involves complex changes where one stage or aspect merges into another. In the first few years most of the changes in posture and movement appear to follow a broad but orderly and reasonably predictable sequence which may be largely due to a dependence on the maturation of the neural system (Wyke, 1975). However, inherited physical characteristics and personal traits, anatomical and physiological growth and maturation, as well as environmental experiences influence the mode of development and performance. Therefore within this broad sequence of development there is a large degree of variability which increases with age (Cratty, 1979). Even within the same infant various aspects of motor development may occur at different rates proceeding rapidly or slowly, starting early or commencing late (Touwen, 1976).

The building blocks for later effective and efficient motor performance are laid down in the first two to three years after birth when the ability to sustain a stable postural background, control movement, balance and co-ordination as well as plan and carry out a desired action are established. A child uses movement to perform and repeat a variety of activities which in turn will promote the development of an efficient interplay of muscle action, strength, flexibility and endurance. Any interference or abnormality of this early development either during the antenatal period or first few years is likely to have adverse effects on the efficiency and skill of movement throughout life. A clear understanding of the developmental changes which occur during this time is therefore essential if one is to recognize problems which lie outside the expected range of normal and then initiate appropriate interventions.

As with all children, those with Down Syndrome have their own unique personalities and characteristics of development. In addition it is likely that they will have some features of the syndrome which adversely influence motor development. Maturational delay in central nervous system organization (Barnet *et al.*, 1971), low muscle tone (Cowie, 1970), and problems within the automatic postural control system (Shumway-Cook and Woollacott, 1985; Haley, 1987), particularly weight shift and body orienting (Shepherd, 1979) and balance (Shumway-Cook and Woollacott, 1985) are some features that have been identified. In addition, delay in walking and differences in the pattern of gait (Lydic and Steele, 1979; Parker and Bronks, 1980) as well as poor posture and obesity are frequently identified as movement difficulties in the population with Down syndrome. Orthopaedic problems, the most serious being joint subluxations and dislocations, may occur as a result of low muscle tone and joint laxity (Diamond *et al.*, 1981; Harris 1984). Structural anomalies particularly the hypoplasia of the odonotoid process allowing subluxation of the atlanto-axial joint of the neck can also lead to major problems (Schiemer and Abroms, 1980). It is clear that the infant with any of these problems can miss achieving some of the essential first phases of motor development or become 'stuck' at a particular stage.

Lack of opportunity to move well will not only adversely affect the quality, strength and endurance of motor performance but is also likely to result in poor feedback and a lack of success-ful achievement, leading to a further reduction in initiative, poor concentration and reduced learning potential. It was suggested by Henderson (1987) that children and young people with Down syndrome do not keep up with their peers in terms of motor development. On the other hand, changes in societal attitudes and expectations, improved health care and dietary control, as well as easier access to experiential opportunities are likely to influence positively each individual's development.

MOTOR DEVELOPMENT: IMPLICATIONS FOR THE CHILD WITH DOWN SYNDROME

The development of movement commences in utero as the foetus grows, changes position, bends and stretches. This movement, which is essential for the development of articulating joints, appears from the eighth week onwards (Wyke, 1975). De Vries *et al.* (1985) recorded by ultra-sound scanning, a variety of patterns of movement from the eighth week after conception onwards. During the second and third in-utero trimesters some of the most remarkable features of brain development occur with the proliferation, migration and differentiation of the neurons. Even though by term (37–42 weeks) the nervous system is normally well developed and capable of complex activities (Holt, 1977) considerable change is still occurring and the neural structures necessary for sensorimotor integration and higher level functions are still immature (Brown, 1974; Freeman and Brann, 1977). Much neural and brain development continues after the baby is born.

Posture and movement after birth

When born at term, the posture of the newborn infant is normally dominated by flexion. The limbs are flexed and adducted towards the midline and traction (holding the two hands and gently raising) will elicit a strong flexor response of the neck and shoulders. Even in the infant born early the flexor components of posture and movement become stronger as the expected due date approaches (Prechtl, 1977; Robinson, 1966). During the few weeks following birth [term] small circular or arc-like limb movements which appear to be spontaneous occur frequently. At this time also a number of reflex patterns of posture and movement can be observed or elicited. These more stereotyped reflex patterns of movement which generally occur in response to a specific stimulus such as touch, pressure, movement or position in relation to gravity, signify that the neurological pathways are defined and intact. A number of these reflex patterns of movement are very useful in the formal assessment of motor development at this age (Paine and Oppe, 1966; Holt, 1977; Prechtl, 1977) but their importance in relation to later development is as yet unresolved.

Posturally, during the first weeks, the infant becomes generally much more extensor in the trunk as well as in the shoulder and pelvic girdle and at times can be quite asymmetrical particularly if lying on the back. The extensor posturing in this position is largely due to the influence of the tonic labyrinthine reflex while the asymmetrical positioning of the limbs is influenced by the asymmetrical tonic neck reflex. The influence of the primitive reflex patterns on the posture and movement of the infant gradually lessens and although still dependent upon support to counteract gravity, definite evidence of head control is soon observed. This head control becomes apparent with the ability to centralize the head to the midline when lying on the back [supine], to lift it up when resting on the tummy and elbows [prone] and to hold it upright with gentle bobbing movements while being supported in sitting. The ability to bring the hands [and feet] together towards the midline to reach for, grasp and hold a toy are soon attained. The achievement of head control makes handling and positioning for bathing, feeding, nursing, and socializing so much easier. Eye to eye contact, a smile, a change of expression and an ability to look around are very important in the life of the baby, parents and extended family.

The newborn behaviour of the infant with Down syndrome may exhibit poor early flexion, immaturity of some reflex posture and movement responses and difficulty in establishing a good nutritive suck-swallow (Cowie, 1970). Head control may be a little slow in developing particularly if low muscle tone is present. This means that handling and positioning during daily activities require special attention. Sometimes the infant with Down syndrome may learn to roll over into supine earlier than expected but rolling onto the tummy may not be achieved for several months (Harris, 1984). Rather than reflecting precocious development this early rolling appears to be associated with a strong preference for lying on the back rather than on the tummy.

Postural orientation and balance

One of the most important stages of motor development is the ability to orientate to gravity and to control the posture of the body in relation to its own position. The infant's ability to adjust to gravity and to movement of its own body becomes apparent through development of the 'righting reactions' (Peiper, 1963; Paine *et al.*, 1964; Bobath and Bobath, 1972). Positive reactions of the head to gravity in both vertical and horizontal positions, Landau response to prone suspension and body-on-body as well as body-on-head righting are normally present by the time the child is ready for sitting, creeping on the tummy and pushing up on to hands and knees (Fiorentino, 1972). Having achieved this basic postural control, infants can interact more positively with their surroundings and soon attempt to move independently around the local environment. Often this is first by rolling but may be by tummy creeping, pushing backwards, swivelling to either side or progressing forward.

At this stage also, when the infant is being supported in standing, there is a strong tendency for bilateral supporting [extending] evidenced by the pleasure of 'bouncing' on the feet but quite soon the ability to shift the weight to one side allowing the other limb to be free to move independently will become apparent. The ability to weight shift, support unilaterally then diagonally and rotate around a stable or fixed point precedes efficient reciprocal creeping or crawling on hands and knees, achieving lying to sitting and pulling to stand. Furthermore the achievement of new positions and activities where the centre of gravity is raised means that the child will need to learn how to maintain the position of choice despite forces and influences which may disturb it.

Parachute and forward, side, or backwards protective ['saving'] reactions are automatic reactions to sudden movement through space or shifts of weight. Equilibrium reactions on the other hand are learned responses counteracting the disturbing force (Palisano, 1988). These compensatory movements occur in response to a need to maintain or regain a desired position. Therefore these learned reactions are acquired after the desired position has been achieved. For example, Burnett and Johnson (1971) reported that equilibrium reactions in standing and walking progressively matured one to six months after independent walking had been achieved. The equilibrium reactions interact harmoniously with the righting reactions to ensure balance and a stable postural background so necessary for consistent performance of efficient motor activities. When these reactions are unsuccessful in retaining balance the protective reactions will once again be used in an effort to 'save' the child from injury. Refinement of balance and skills learning proceeds throughout childhood.

In the infant with Down syndrome, delay in the development of head and body righting is a difficulty frequently noted (Cowie, 1970; Haley, 1987) while Lydic and Steele (1979) reported the lack of rotation along the central axis of the body in those infants who presented with abnormal patterns of sitting and walking. It has been suggested that this lack of normal righting reactions could be the reason for the tendency in children with Down syndrome to 'flip over', rather than roll smoothly (Harris, 1984), and for the unusual way in which many infants with Down syndrome achieve sitting. A frequently observed tendency to move from prone into sitting by widely abducting the legs then pushing on the arms until the bottom is behind the hips and stable for sitting has been described in detail by Lydic and Steele (1979).

Haley (1986, 1987) investigated the emergence of the automatic postural reactions [righting, protective, and equilibrium] in a group of infants with Down syndrome compared with a developmentally matched group of non-Down syndrome infants. The relationship of postural reactions to chronological age was less strong and a difference in sequence [protective reactions appearing relatively earlier] was reported in the infants with Down syndrome. The association between postural reactions and motor milestones, however, was similar in both groups even though the rate of development differed. Instead of looking at the developmental presentation of postural and balance reactions, Shumway-Cook and Woollacott (1985) examined the development of neural control processes underlying stance balance in both children with Down syndrome and children who did not have Down syndrome. This study has important implications for the treatment of balance problems in these children because it showed that, although externally produced perturbations to balance using a hydraulically controlled platform showed that onset latencies of postural muscles in the children with Down syndrome were significantly slower than in the children without Down syndrome, myotatic latencies in both groups were similar. This suggests that balance problems may not be due to hypotonia i.e. a decreased segmental neuron pool excitability and stretch reflex mechanism, but are rather a result of defects or differences within higher level postural control mechanisms.

These authors recommended that remediation of balance should focus on motor co-ordination by improving the way in which multiple muscle groups effectively and efficiently act together and by improving planning mechanisms which adapt postural response patterns to changing tasks and performance needs. They continued by reminding readers that neither of these processes is voluntary or conscious, stating that 'Maintenance of stability requires the execution of fast [automatic] postural responses with onset latencies below those of voluntary reaction time responses' (Shumway-Cook and Woollacott, 1985, p. 1321). Although a number of writings refer to a problem of balance experienced by children with Down syndrome, it is clear that the major problem lies in the components of balance which are postural righting, weight shift and support, awareness of position in space and the strength and co-ordination of appropriate equilibrium reactions.

It is highly likely that delay in attaining and subsequent inefficiency of postural stability in children with Down syndrome is an important factor in the timing of the achievement of the motor milestones of sitting up, crawling and walking. Shepherd (1979) considered that an inability to weight shift and ineffective body orienting and balance were instrumental in causing the infant with Down syndrome to get 'stuck' in certain positions such as wide based long sitting. An inability to weight shift and rotate around the body axis could also adversely affect the development of playing with toys while lying prone, creeping, crawling, moving from one position to another [e.g. sit to hands and knees and reverse], pulling to stand through half-kneeling, cruising and walking. A lack of dynamic co-contraction of the trunk postural muscles however means that forwards or sideways self support mechanisms through the arms, may be necessary for a longer than normal period. This is likely to delay the development of transference and play using two hands.

Even when sitting allows both hands to be free there is often a delay in the establishment of a pincer and opposition grasp and index pointing. Furthermore the co-ordination of two hands in manipulative activities requires a degree of postural control and stability around the shoulders. The implications are wider, as the learning and efficient performance of both gross and fine motor skills including good co-ordinated lip closure and firm jaw action required for drinking and eating, depend upon the automatic control of background posture. But not all delay is due to poor postural and balance mechanisms. It has been noted clinically that in sitting, shortness of the upper limbs frequently reduces the infant's ability to use the arms for support or for sideways stability. Poor muscle tone and strength and joint hypermobility have all been implicated as possible causes of abnormal and delayed motor development.

Sensori-motor aspects

Once the child can explore the local environment tactilely, visually, auditorily and through movement [proprioceptively], then the integration of all of these inputs starts to give the infant/child a sense of awareness in that environment. The importance of sensation in development particularly in the control and peformance of movement has been identified by numerous authors (Twitchell, 1954; Clark *et al.*, 1977; Goodkin, 1980). In 1977, Holt described rather simply the emergence of sensory awareness as a succession of stages. In the early stages [three to four months] the infant tends to be preoccupied with one single sensory channel at a time to the exclusion of other input. As this stage passes, there is an increasing tendency to use more than one sense for a task, followed by the flexibility to switching from one channel to another or using simultaneously two or more senses for different tasks. This integration and co-ordination of functions enhances the ability to adapt a response to the specific needs of the time, to interpret feedback regarding success or failure of the efforts and to provide the basis for learning by experience. The senses of touch, joint position and movement, movement through space [vestibular] as well as the special senses of vision and hearing all combine to provide children with a sense and awareness of self as well as a means of interpreting and learning about the world around them.

Grasp and manipulation of objects in the hands utilize the integration of sensation and feedback in the development of co-ordinated and purposeful actions. The hands and upper limbs also play a very important role in the development of everyday functional activities. As with other aspects of development there is a general sequence or progression (Erhardt, 1974). The initial grasp reflex [strong finger flexion] is replaced first by finger plucking/clutching until a grasp in the palm can be achieved. The object in the palm is then gradually grasped more radially until the thumb and base of the first finger can be used in a pincer action. Concurrently the infant starts to use the flat hand to pat or 'feel' different textures. The gross pincer action becomes more refined as the thumb moves up the index finger gradually applying pressure more and more distally. As a climax the thumb is then rotated so that the pads of the thumb and index finger are opposed allowing tiny objects to be picked up and rolled or felt (Touwen, 1971). Index pointing and index 'sensing' appear at this stage also and play an essential role in the development and interpretation of sensation.

Use of hands in simple functional activities is an important aspect of early motor development. The ability to pick up very small objects is usually achieved several months before release is controlled thus the tendency to 'give' but keep holding the object is a common stage of pre-release development. Not only are hold and release important for function and play but also the ability to rotate the forearm, that is, to turn the hand over. Keeping the spoon in the same plane during the early stage of self feeding is the reason why half of the spoonful tips down the chest rather than into the open mouth. During this period the average child will use the tips of the tripod three fingers for the more delicate operations but resort to a palmar grasp for more forceful projects. Soon after, an ability to screw and unscrew not only allows a greater range of activities and experiences but can be an ability which will lead to danger such as opening doors and taking lids off forbidden containers.

In reporting the milestones for children with Down syndrome, Cunningham (1982) listed a number of items which required a level of sensori-motor integration as well as fine grasp and motor co-ordination. Items involving a sense of space and object permanence were shown as somewhat delayed in their achievement but it is not known if the major factor was the lack of motor co-ordination, a delayed development of sensori-motor integration or a combination of both. As a result of a study comparing sensory evoked EEG responses, Barnet *et al.* (1971) suggested that infants/children with Down syndrome appeared to have some maturational delay in central nervous system organization leading to a deficiency in ability to adapt to and moderate the response to repetitive input. McDade and Adler (1980) reported that the children they studied had difficulties with storage and processing of both visual and auditory input. Obviously many factors contribute to the development of, as well as a delay in, the performance of fine and sensori-motor skills. Most programmes of early intervention appear to include activities designed to enhance sensori-motor integration, organization, and feedback necessary for modification and adaptation of motor action (Hughes, 1971; Harris, 1980; 1981; 1988).

Locomotion and motor independence

Independence in walking, ability to grasp and release and explore objects, as well as the integration of various sensory inputs, awareness of the permanence of objects and a desire to actively participate in the environment opens the way for a widening of horizons and the learning of new skills. As the child proceeds into and through various stages there is not only a refinement of balance, co-ordination, gait, hand function and an appreciation of the space and shape of objects but also a desire to make things happen. Piaget (Flavell, 1963) called this a period of experimentation.

Bipedal locomotion and the maintenance of an erect posture are key elements of development during this period. As indicated previously, an ability to orientate to gravity and the development of weight shift and support are important for the achievement of independent walking. This means that the child must be able to shift weight to one side, and the limb thus taking the extra load should be able to support the body weight. This involves dynamic muscle co-contraction in the supporting leg while the muscles of the non-loadbearing limb are in 'active' mode, allowing freedom of movement for stepping forward (Stockmeyer, 1980).

In the early phase of walking the child has no or very poorly developed equilibrium reactions so only partial weight shift on to the supporting leg may occur and then the free leg may be only partially relaxed to step, hence the tendency for a stiff legged, wide based gait. Stooping, squatting, standing up from the floor, kneel standing and climbing are all activities practised by the child which provide experience in mid range joint/muscle control. Balance in standing involves a complex integration of signals from proprioceptive [muscle and joint], visual and vestibular systems and a need to retain the desired position against disturbing forces (O'Connell and Gardiner, 1972; Cody and Nelson, 1978). Balance is more than an ability to stay upright but is a dynamic process that is continually being refined in response to a need. The equilibrium reactions and the ability to rotate around the central axis of the body become evident once the child has achieved each new major position such as sitting, crawling, kneeling, standing and walking. Before a child can develop efficiency in functional balance, an ability to step forward with each leg, have a narrow base as in the more mature gait, and to progress up and down the stairs, it is necessary for good equilibrium reactions in standing and during walking to be established. About 12 months after learning to walk, most children have a gait pattern similar to that of an adult in that there is an initial heel strike, weight shift forward along the foot and thrust from the base of the toes. At this time, however, they have a short, quick, jerky stride and considerable associated body movement (Burnett and Johnson 1971). The gait gradually improves in efficiency and flow over a period of three or more years.

Children learning to jump, run, throw, catch and kick a ball are experiencing a period of training in motor control, balance, spring/propulsion, rhythm, strength, endurance and energy efficiency. According to Espenschade and Eckert (1980), the toddler and preschool period is the time when basic locomotor patterns are perfected and a variety of hand co-ordinations are learned. Functional motor control tends to commence proximally [at hips and shoulders as observed in early stages of catching or kicking a ball, riding a trike or drawing] and proceeds distally until isolated movements can be performed allowing mastery of fine motor skills. Writing with a pencil, cutting with scissors and other fine motor skills involve not only highly tuned motor control of fingers and wrists so well described by Rosenbloom and Horton (1971) and Holle (1976) but also a degree of perceptual awareness of space, position, movement and symbols.

The child with Down syndrome may achieve independent walking any time from the first birthday onwards, but sometimes not until four years or more. An immaturity of the gait pattern is a commonly recognized feature in children with Down syndrome and a number of factors which could delay or interfere with the quality of bipedal locomotion have been identified. Parker and Bronks (1980) analysed the gait of six and seven year old children with Down syndrome and described a general immaturity but wide developmental range, a tendency to contact the floor with the whole or flat foot rather than a heel-toe mechanism, and poor motor control of the distal segments. This latter statement was supported not only by poor dorsiflexion at the ankles but also by a lack of normal wrist extension. These authors suggested a high energy cost due to the immaturity and inefficiency of the gait mechanism.

It has been suggested that children, adolescents and adults with Down syndrome perform less well than chronological age peers in terms of physical fitness and motor performance such as ball skills (Reid, 1987). Unfortunately, due to a paucity of objective information it is difficult to establish if this is a problem related to a lack of opportunity, immaturity of motor ability, or both.

ASSESSMENT

Infants and children who are 'at risk' or who present with delays or difficulties in motor development require a comprehensive assessment of all aspects of motor development to reveal both areas of strength as well as areas of difficulty or abnormality. In addition to the use of a standardized developmental test, the physiotherapist uses a criterion based assessment which views motor development both qualitatively as well as quantitatively in terms of age-related gross and fine motor abilities and function, postural control, balance and co-ordination, the capacity to adapt to change and the ability to learn skills. The basis for the development of these competencies lies in the integrity of the neurological, muscle and skeletal systems as well as the ability to receive, integrate and process [interpret] the intrinsic and extrinsic input in the selection, processing and control of motor output. Evaluation of all of these aspects therefore involves a keen observation of posture, movement and performance during a number of preselected tasks and activities as well as testing specifically, according to standardized procedures and set criteria, of neurological, muscle and skeletal, postural and sensori-motor functioning (Rogers, 1987).

Assessment which 'rates' or puts a value on particular actions or responses of the constantly changing developing infant or child consequently is not a simple task but a dynamic, complex and multifaceted activity. Due to this complexity, the assessor should avoid the trap of trying to assess too many aspects in great detail thus fatiguing the child and obtaining an inaccurate result (Burns *et al.*, 1989). It is important to choose an assessment which clearly evaluates all aspects with the minimum of fuss and time yet encourages and allows children to show optimum performance. The skill of the assessor not only lies in the competency to perform the specified testing procedures but also in the ability to develop a rapport of respect and trust with the child and parents. Even under the most stringent criteria and conducive environment, an assessment can only reveal the particular attributes or problems as expressed at that point in time and under the conditions which prevail during the assessment. For example, the time of day in relation to meal or sleep times, travel prior to the assessment, the basic health and feelings of well-being on that particular day can markedly influence performance in some or all of the test items.

Emphasis has been placed on the assessment of the infant and young child but the importance of an accurate and comprehensive assessment does not diminish as the child grows older into adolescence and adulthood. Like other elderly persons in the community, the elderly person with Down Syndrome also has special needs. The overall aims of an assessment remain the same but age-appropriate techniques, equipment and tasks must be used.

Assessment procedure

Before commencing the assessment it is important to ensure that the time of the day is appropriate, i.e., not sleep or mealtime, that one or both parents (or familiar caregiver) is present, that it is in an environment which is warm, friendly and age-appropriate in terms of its furniture, surroundings and appealing equipment, and that all requirements for the actual testing are strategically located. It is recommended that an assessment should commence with a period of observation of motor ability and function. The parent should be urged to interact with the infant or child and in play to encourage motor activity and/or function. If older children or adults are being assessed then they may wish to have a friend present. At all times it is imperative to respect, in all undertakings, the client being assessed as well as any attending persons.

A period of observation at the commencement of an assessment is extremely important as it provides the physiotherapist with the opportunity to observe not only what the child can and cannot do but also the quality of the performance, and the ability to initiate interaction with or respond to a familiar person. This time also acts as an 'ice breaker' making it easier for the assessor to become part of the activity and, as a stranger, to enter into the child's personal space. The order in which the more formal testing proceeds depends on the age and co-operation of the infant/child or older client. Nonetheless it is always preferable to undertake the least threatening tests (those not involving handling) first, then those which cause the least anxiety and finally those which involve unfamiliar positions or procedures. This latter group would include tests of tone, range of movement, strength, postural righting, equilibrium, and the sensori-motor test of vestibular function. Successful assessment depends on more than the assessor's ability to observe accurately, to test correctly in accordance with the procedure and criteria of the evaluation, and to interpret discerningly. It depends also on skills of communication, an ability to gain and maintain interest and co-operation, the avoidance of boredom, frustration or feelings of failure, and thus the promotion of the child's 'best' effort. A negative experience in a formal assessment can undermine the confidence of both the child/adult and the parent or friend.

INTERVENTION: PRINCIPLES AND GUIDELINES

Movement is fun! Through movement the child explores, plays, interacts, functions and learns. In other words the child both learns to move and moves to learn. Infants, young children, adolescents and adults who have difficulty in movement usually present with a combination of competencies as well as problems. Using knowledge of the development, mechanisms, control and adaptability of movement, the physiotherapist aims to optimize the strengths and overcome the problems of each individual. It is important, however, to recognize the limitations of intervention as many of the motor differences presenting in those with Down syndrome are due to basic anomalies in the central nervous and musculoskeletal systems, which cannot be changed (Harris, 1988). Gibson and Harris (1988) recommended that 'intervention curricula [should] reflect the unique biological and behavioural properties of the syndrome, taking into account the individual differences which are independent of the etiological label' (p. 1).

From the time of birth, advice to parents regarding feeding, handling and interacting with their infant can assist both the parent and infant to overcome some early anxieties and problems. During parent/caregiver-infant interaction it is possible to draw the attention of the adult to the positive aspects of the baby's development while also stressing the importance of gaining and holding attention. Progressively more specific positioning, handling and stimulation (Lydic and Steele, 1979; Harris 1981, 1988) can be used to enhance the normal automatic postural and movement responses during daily care activities carried out by the parent/care-giver. Thus bathing, eating, and changing times become activities that promote positive aspects of posture and movement control, while during play and quiet times encouragement of eye contact not only enhances early social interaction but assists in the development of postural alignment. From the beginning, muscle action is improved through appropriate activity and once sensory integration starts to develop, co-ordination of eye and hand, hand and hand, as well as other limb movements can be encouraged.

Although stimulation and facilitation of automatic responses have a role to play, it is essential to recognize the importance of introducing early the appropriate challenges for self achievement. Encouragement to try and to keep trying is needed often but whenever possible the opportunity for self initiative and achievement should be presented. There is nothing like success to inspire the achiever to repeat the performance. The importance of learning through experience and repetition underlies most programmes (Harris, 1984).

Through careful and comprehensive assessment, the physiotherapist not only ascertains immature movement patterns and the motor problems interfering with development but also identifies the strengths of the child and plans treatment programmes accordingly. Due to the varying presentation of aspects of Down syndrome, together with the variability of development itself and the personal characteristics of each child, most programmes of intervention need to be individually tailored. The importance of close collaboration between all professionals and caregivers in deciding on goals and objectives and in the formulation of a programme which recognizes individual needs has been emphasised by Hughes (1971), Harris (1980) and Gibson and Harris (1988). The professionals likely to be involved in the very early phase of development include a physiotherapist, a speech therapist, a paediatrician, and within a few months an occupational therapist and an early childhood special educator.

The daily life of the infant and young child, however, is in the home so the parents and caregivers have a unique and integral role in any intervention. To fill this role, they require a good understanding of the specific aims of each aspect of the programme, its goals or expected response, and the methods that can be used to achieve the desired outcome. Many parents need emotional support as well as information and understanding of 'how' to help their child (Mitchell, 1979; Cunningham and Glenn, 1987) and therefore the art of working with parents and meeting their individual needs must be developed. In analysing the effects of early intervention Gunn and Berry (1989) suggested that 'professionals tend to divorce themselves from the social ecology of early intervention.' They continued that in emphasizing the skills to be taught to others the professionals may 'fail to examine their own role and influence', (p. 240). It is clear that all professionals working with parents need to take a realistic and common sense view with the focus clearly on the child and family, and not on the programme or any specific aspect of intervention.

As children enter school and progress into adolescence they are more involved in their own decision making and the classroom teacher and physical educator/instructor plays a major role in providing programmes of education and activity. Parents together with therapist and medical advisers still have an important role and the need for consultation and collaboration does not diminish.

3

Activities during infancy

Sue Price and Rose-Anne Kelso

INTRODUCTION

Many babies with Down syndrome have poor muscle tone and lie quietly in their cots so not attracting attention with their movements and vocalizations to the same extent as other children. For this reason, there is a tendency for caregivers to think that they are 'good' babies and leave them to lie peacefully in their cots. Yet the optimal development of these children relies on their opportunities to learn about themselves and their environment. The day-to-day interactions between the babies and their caregivers can provide handling and play experiences which make an essential contribution to these learning opportunities.

Handling and playing activities help all infants to become more aware of their own bodies, their physical and social environments, and the relationships between them. Many babies with Down syndrome need not only these general experiences but also specific activities that will help them to experience the feelings of normal movement.

The following sections describe some movement activities that are relevant for babies with Down syndrome. Once a movement has been developed, it should be practised, so that it becomes an established part of the infant's movement repertoire. Care must be taken not to tire the infant and a little activity often is the best guide. This is especially true for babies with heart problems as they are more susceptible to tiring. It is also important that the activities remain enjoyable and not a source of stress for either caregiver or baby.

The activities are presented as ideas for physiotherapists and caregivers and are not to be regarded as a treatment programme. The global term caregiver, rather than mother or parent, has been used as most of the activities can be undertaken by any person caring for the child. Indeed it would be advantageous for the baby if everyone who acted as caregiver, whether sibling, grandparent, aunt, uncle, or nanny, adopted these practices when interacting with the child.

It is hoped that the activities will be adapted so that they become part of the normal day-to-day interactions with the baby. The most common day-to-day routines are those involved with feeding, changing, bathing, and dressing. These functional routines include handling, lifting and carrying and each offers the opportunity for playful interactions between the infant and the caregiver. The activities are suggested as part of these normal daily interctions with the baby.

The suggestions should be considered as guidelines and as showing basic principles so that the activities may be extended to include other techniques by interested therapists.

FEEDING

Problems with feeding are not uncommon in babies with Down syndrome, possibly because of hypotonicity of the orofacial muscles and the small mouth structure. To make feeding easier, stimulation in and around the mouth may be used to improve the sensitivity of the muscles of the face, mouth, neck and tongue. Also, the caregiver should take time to experiment with the more comfortable and practical feeding positions.

If the baby is bottle fed, the infant should be supported in a half sitting position. If the mother is breastfeeding, she can achieve active control of the baby's head and mouth by holding the back of the baby's head with one hand, while leaving the other hand free to stimulate lip closure and sucking if necessary. As always, it is important to ensure that the rest of the baby's body is supported appropriately (Figure 3.1).

The mother may find at times that she needs to give her baby more 'breathing space' by changing to a less encompassing position.

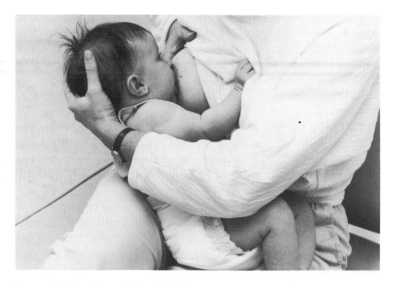

Figure 3.1 Position during feeding.

If the baby has difficulty in closing the lips tightly around the teat or nipple, the muscles may need to be stimulated before feeding. This can be done by stroking around the corners of the baby's mouth with a finger. One corner of the mouth is stimulated first through the arc of a semi-circle from the top lip to the bottom lip. After waiting two or three seconds for a response, the other corner of the mouth should be stroked in a similar fashion. The baby will usually respond with a slight puckering of the lips although for some babies, the stimulation increases awareness without a visible response.

The stroking should be repeated two or three times on each side of the mouth. This technique can be repeated any time during feeding or when the baby stops to rest. Care must be taken, however, to avoid over-stimulation which may distract the baby's attention from feeding or even cause fatigue.

When bottle feeding, if the baby tends to gag, check the size of the teat. A smaller teat may be more appropriate.

If the baby thrusts out the tongue when attempting to feed, the tip of the tongue should be lightly touched with the caregiver's finger. The caregiver should then wait for the baby to respond by retracting the tongue. With a small percentage of babies, this procedure is not effective. In such cases, the tongue could be gently pushed down behind the bottom gum.

These 'tongue tipping' techniques can be repeated any time during the day to help stimulate tongue mobility. Good tongue mobility is essential for good oral development throughout life.

Once the tongue is retracted, the teat can be placed in the baby's mouth. It should be placed on the top of the tongue and not pushed back against a bent up tongue or under the tongue as the baby will not be able to suck properly in these circumstances.

There are a number of techniques which the caregiver may try in feeding the baby. For example, in order to achieve a firmer seal, the ring and index fingers of the hand holding the bottle can gently push the corners of the baby's mouth against the teat or nipple. This will help to prevent the baby sucking in air and dribbling from the side of the mouth (Figure 3.2).

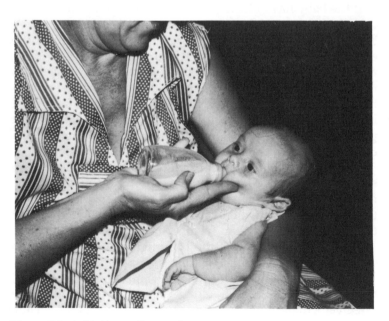

Figure 3.2 Achieving a firm seal.

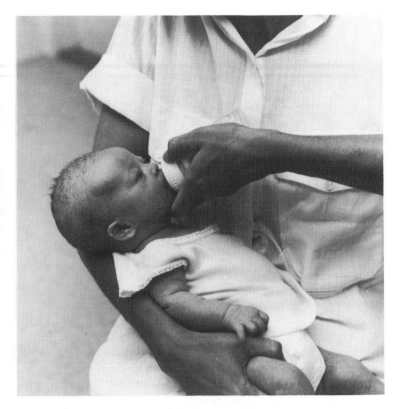

Figure 3.3 Index finger placed to aid swallowing.

To aid swallowing, the index finger can be placed under the baby's chin. Care must be taken not to place the finger too far back as this may cause the baby to gag. Figure 3.3 shows the correct position with the finger just behind the bony area of the jaw. Figure 3.4 shows an incorrect position with the finger too far back.

If the baby has a poor lip seal across the top and bottom of the teat, the index and middle fingers may be placed above and below the lips, lightly pressing them together to help lip closure. Figure 3.5 is a photograph that has been taken without the bottle so that the finger position may be seen clearly, but the bottle should be held in the other hand.

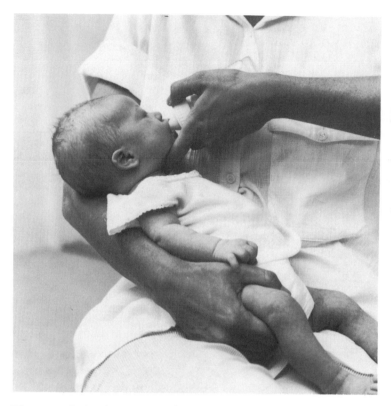

Figure 3.4 Index finger is too far back.

To improve the baby's sucking ability, intermittent traction can be applied to the bottle. This can be achieved by gently pulling the bottle until the teat moves about 1 cm within the baby's mouth. The traction is then released so that the baby sucks the teat back in. This is repeated rhythmically as the baby sucks. This technique is completed gently so that the caregiver can feel at all times that the baby has 'hold' of the teat. Once again, the infant should be given time to respond to the stimulus.

Any combination of these techniques can be used at each feed and they should be continued until the baby can cope without them. This may take a few hours, a few weeks, or a few months. The caregiver should be encouraged to experiment in a search for the most appropriate combination.

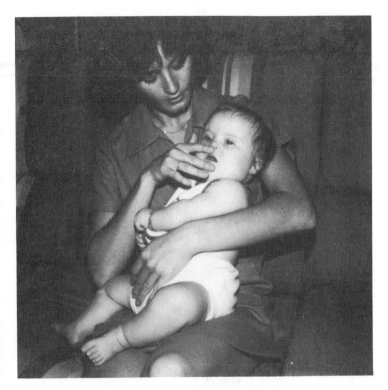

Figure 3.5 Showing position of fingers for a better lip seal.

When starting to feed the baby with solid foods, a spoon which is short, shallow, and rounded should be used. A small amount of food should be placed on the front of the spoon to make it easier for the baby to cope. The spoon should be placed on top of the tongue and guided into the mouth, especially if the tongue is not resting on the floor of the mouth. If the tongue is not well positioned, the tongue tipping exercises described previously may be used.

It is important that the caregiver should not passively remove the contents of the spoon by pushing up against the roof of the mouth or the top gum to scrape off the food. By applying gentle pressure on the tongue with the spoon, the baby will be encouraged to loosen the mouth and actively remove the food with the inside of the lips. Again, it is important to allow the baby time to respond.

If the baby has poor lip closure, the techniques described previously for bottle feeding can be used before feeding. Slight pressure can be given behind the chin if the infant finds it difficult to swallow.

When the baby is ready to start chewing, a small amount of solid food such as meat or crust can be placed between the molar gums and cheek on one side of the mouth. This stimulates the chewing action and the baby uses the tongue to manipulate the food into the centre of the mouth for swallowing. This will further develop tongue tone and movement.

During the early days of introducing solids, the messiness of mealtimes can be used to stimulate lip and tongue movement.

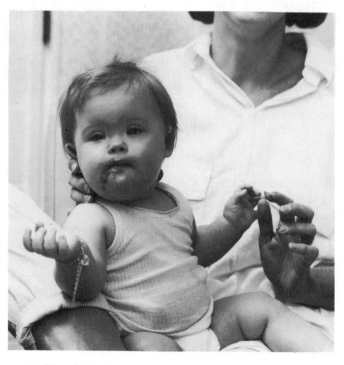

Figure 3.6 Stimulating tongue movement.

Babies can be encouraged to use their tongues to retrieve food from their faces. Substances that need a lot of work to clear the mouth, for example, a teaspoonful of peanut butter (paste) can be used.

CARRYING

All babies are carried but it is especially important that the baby with Down syndrome be carried and handled frequently during the first few weeks and months. The infant needs the general stimulation of handling which occurs during carrying, and also during carrying specific stimuli to facilitate the development of head and postural control may be offered.

To encourage the development of postural control, enough head and trunk support should be provided for safety but some freedom should be allowed in order to stimulate babies toward trying to achieve control themselves. The method of carrying the baby should be varied so that the infant experiences different positions, movements, and visual stimuli.

One method is to carry the baby with the infant's stomach and chest along the caregiver's arm. This encourages the

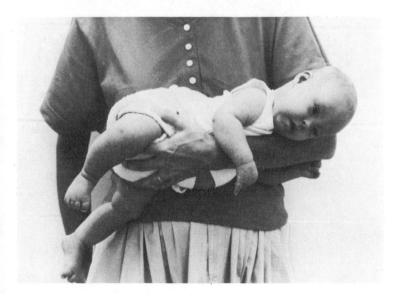

Figure 3.7 An early carrying position.

development of head control and it can be used before head control is achieved. This position is excellent as it allows the baby to see and it encourages good visual interaction and active head movement. Carrying in this way can be achieved with the baby's head either on the hand or at the elbow, depending on comfort and the amount of support needed. The elbow position is shown in Figure 3.7.

Another carrying position that may be used from birth is one in which the baby, though not having head control, will be able to interact with the caregiver. In this position, the infant's head and shoulder are supported in the caregiver's elbow, with the hand of the same arm holding the child's outside leg. This leaves the other arm free (Figure 3.8).

By holding the baby in this semi-sitting position, both head control and visual interaction with the social and physical environment are encouraged. As the child develops some head and postural control, the support may be lowered until only the lower back and pelvis are supported. As more head and back control develops, the support may be reduced even

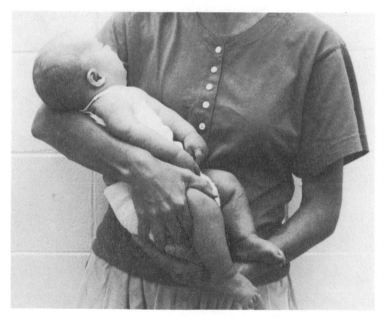

Figure 3.8 Another early carrying position.

further to the pelvis only. As babies gain better back control, even less support is necessary and they can sit comfortably on the caregiver's forearm without the need for back support (Figure 3.9).

Some caregivers prefer to carry the child over the shoulder. While in this position, gently stroking the child's lower back and shoulders may encourage the infant to hold the head up and in the midline.

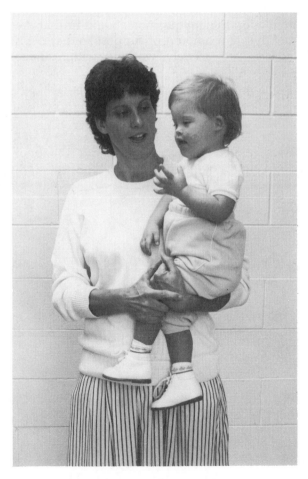

Figure 3.9 Sitting when no back support is required.

Another useful carrying method is on the hip, facing the child outwards, with legs hanging down. In this position, support can be given with one arm in front of the chest and shoulder. Here the child's head is placed in an almost vertical position, minimizing the effect of gravity and allowing ease of head control. Holding the child in this fashion encourages a total extension pattern of the trunk which is important for further development of postural control. This method provides an easy progression to the facilitation of protective extension in the upper limbs.

Other ways may be found for holding or carrying the child. The aim in adopting any position should be that the child is given just the right amount of support so that the neck and back muscles are actively working within their current

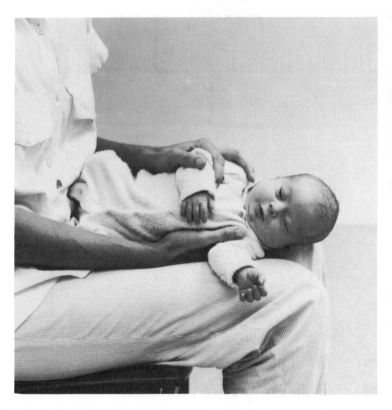

Figure 3.10 How to lift baby from a lying position: stage 1.

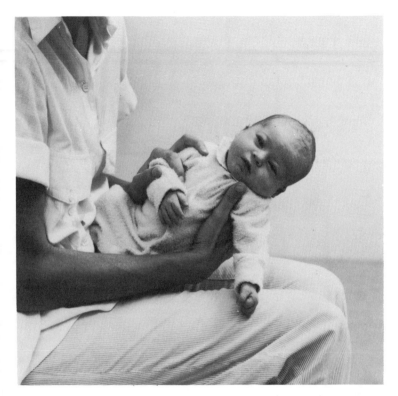

Figure 3.11 Stage 2.

capabilities. No one position is suitable for all situations during the day so it is best to use a position that is appropriate for the specific task or situation. A tired child will always need more support than one who is actively interested in the surroundings. It is also advisable to vary the position from one side to another to avoid postural asymmetry.

LIFTING UP

There are many ways to lift the baby from a lying position. All of them are correct if they incorporate the basic principles of active head control and trunk rotation. Again

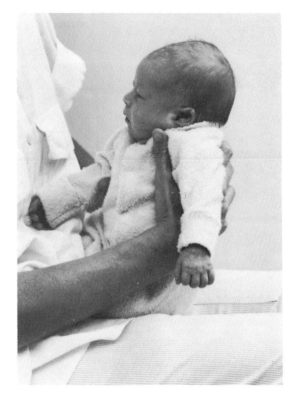

Figure 3.12 Stage 3.

it must be noted that the child should always be handled in a way which will encourage as much head control as possible.

As can be seen from Figures 3.10 to 3.12, direct head support need not be given to even the youngest of babies. As demonstrated, the head and neck support is coming from the left shoulder which in turn is being controlled by the caregiver's right hand. The starting position with the baby on the lap is shown in Figure 3.10. The mid position (Figure 3.11) shows the amount of trunk rotation and the support of the head coming indirectly from the shoulder. If the baby is hypotonic, the whole of the lower trunk may need to be supported as well. Figure 3.12 shows the child about to be lifted for carrying.

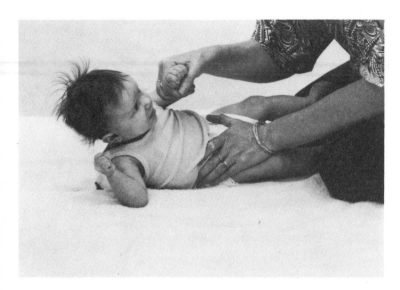

Figure 3.13 Another way to lift baby: stage 1.

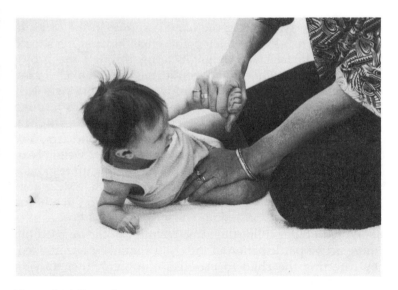

Figure 3.14 Stage 2.

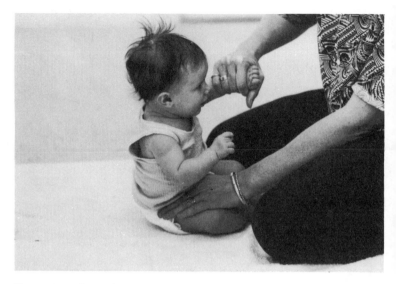

Figure 3.15 Stage 3.

Another way of lifting the baby is shown in the series of Figures 3.13 to 3.15. The main point is that the caregiver should remember to facilitate weight bearing through the baby's supporting arm, while giving gentle traction to the other arm. This method of sitting may be introduced at a surprisingly early age, but the importance of giving the child time to respond must be stressed.

The baby should *not* be just pulled up by one arm. The caregiver should allow time for the gentle traction, weight bearing and rotation to initiate, in the child, a sitting up response. The child can then be gently helped to achieve the sitting position. This is another illustration of trunk rotation in a lifting sequence.

With an older child, the same techniques can be used but more active participation of the child should be encouraged, by directing the child to prop on one hand, then to shift weight and rotate the trunk to that side, using the abdominal muscles.

INCREASING AWARENESS

Sensation is the basis of experience and most children will seek their own sensory stimulation although some must be helped to see, taste, smell, hear, feel, and experience normal movement. In the early postnatal months, the tactile, proprioceptive and vestibular systems contribute most input for the infant to attain and maintain a stable relationship with gravity and the supporting surface.

The development of a body image and of form perception stems from the growth of awareness of the self and of objects in the environment. To help to improve the baby's awareness of the body, firm decisive handling should always be used. Presentation of different objects, people, and positions can help

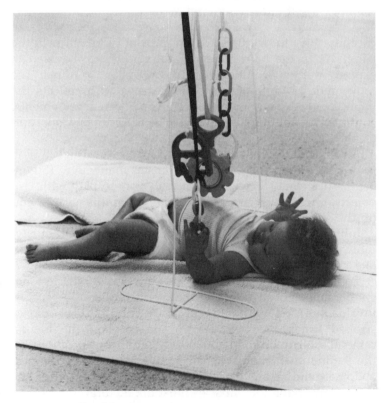

Figure 3.16 Reaching for toys.

to show relationships with others and with space. From an early age, a variety of experiences can be presented to help to stimulate all the senses. As the baby spends more time awake, the activities can be incorporated into play for longer periods of time.

Toys and mobiles that are bright and/or make a sound help to stimulate the baby's eye, head and limb movements. The baby should be encouraged to focus on and visually follow a moving object. The caregiver's face or a bright eye-catching object may be used for the baby to follow. The object can be moved smoothly and slowly in all directions at a distance that is comfortable for the baby to focus.

Soon the baby will start showing an interest in reaching for objects. This may be regarded as a sign of an interest in physically exploring and determining the relationship between the baby's self and the environment.

A commercially available or a home made toy rack is an excellent way to put toys within the sight and reach of the baby. When the baby is ready, the hands will be used to explore the environment aided by vision to direct the movements. Mouthing also will be seen as it reflects the infant's early exploration of objects. As part of a developmental continuum, mouthing should soon be replaced by visual and tactile exploration.

A baby will reach with one hand for an object (Figure 3.17) then take it with the other in a transfer manoeuvre (Figure 3.18). After this stage, the baby will start to play with two objects, one in each hand. The ability to do this will depend on the size and shape of the object.

Initially the grasp will tend to be in the palm. Gradually, more use of the thumb will be noted followed by a more pincer-like action between the thumb and the side of the index finger.

To increase the baby's body awareness and muscle tone, gentle massage all over the body, including the face, is invaluable. The length of the arms, body and legs should be stroked firmly but lightly with the palm of the hands, remembering to do so in both supine and prone positions. In the supine position, stroke diagonally across the chest and abdomen starting at the neck and finishing down the opposite thigh. The abdominal muscles must not be forgotten as they are important for moving from lying to sitting as well as for

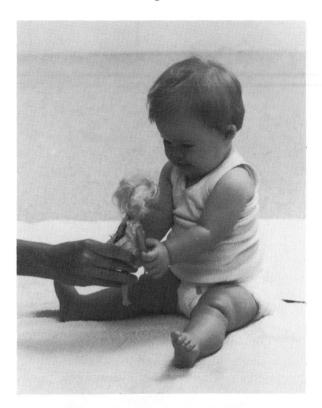

Figure 3.17 Reaching and transferring to other hand.

their role in trunk stability. With an older baby, it is possible to use games like 'see saw marjory daw' in which the movements used can elicit abdominal muscle contraction.

In the prone position, stroke longitudinally from shoulder to thighs especially around the scapula muscles. The stroking in the prone position will assist forearm propping.

When the baby is in the supine position, by using *very gentle* compression, proprioceptive input may help increase muscle contraction and sensory awareness of position and movement. With the joints in an anatomically stable position, this input can be given through the upper limbs by giving gentle pressure down through the bent arm. In the lower limbs, the input may

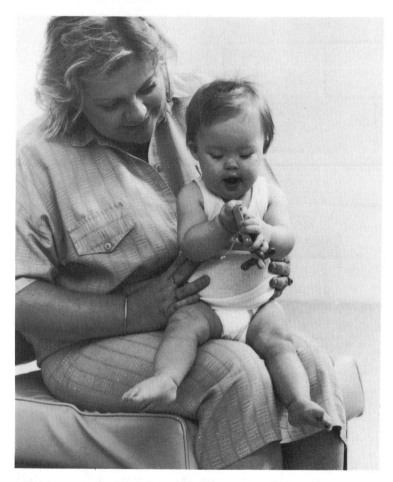

Figure 3.18 Process completed.

be given by applying *gentle* pressure with the heel of the hand
against the baby's heel towards the knee (Figure 3.19).

As voluntary movement starts to develop, this activity can
be extended to encourage kicking. With the baby lying supine,
the lower leg and foot can be grasped and moved alternately
in a kicking or bicycling movement. When the leg is fully
flexed, the caregiver can give an extra pressure through the
heel and then wait momentarily for the baby to try and push
back into the caregiver's hands.

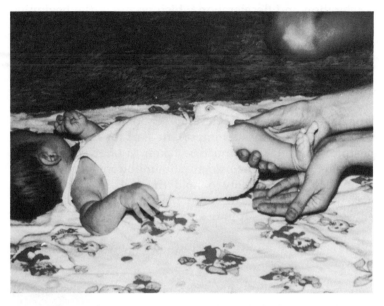

Figure 3.19 Applying gentle pressure through the baby's heel.

The baby's hands can be clapped together to provide movement experience in the midline and to promote shared enjoyment. This will often motivate voluntary activity. Clapping feet together and bringing them up to the mouth will enable the child to visualize as well as to feel the movement of the legs. These common playful activities provide many benefits for the baby.

Initially, the vestibular system is very sensitive to movement. A general reaction when nursing a baby is to rock the infant from side to side. This slow rhythmic movement has a soothing effect on the vestibular system and will often calm a baby and even put the child to sleep. A more 'stimulating' movement can be used to activate the vestibular system. This movement should be smooth and not too fast as over-stimulation can cause fear and uncontrolled postural responses. Moving the baby through space, up in the air, or slowly in a circle while holding the baby out from your chest, are useful activities. Movement to music is very pleasant for both caregivers and children. It should be borne in mind that the angular acceleration and deceleration which occurs at the beginning and end of movement are the most stimulating. Again, little and often is the best rule.

HEAD CONTROL

From a very early age, the development of head control should be encouraged as it is an important start for movement and postural control. Care must be taken to offer suport when necessary. At the same time, it is important not to under-estimate the baby's ability to 'hold' the head, even though this may be momentary. The prone position is very helpful as it encourages elbow support and head lift. The baby should

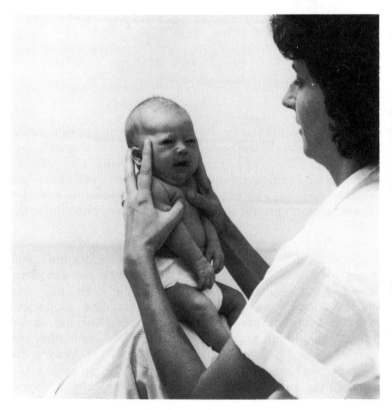

Figure 3.20 Encouraging head control.

experience a variety of positions, however, in order to encourage further development of head control.

For the very floppy baby, initial head control can be encouraged with the baby in a sitting position (Figure 3.20). The head and shoulders should be supported and, if necessary, the side of the trunk also. The palm of the hands should be used to give this support.

When the baby is steady in this position, the support should be moved to about 2 cm from the head while the baby is gently swayed from side to side. The head will move from one side to another but the support will stop the head from moving too far. This is an easier position for gaining initial head control even when the trunk still needs full support.

The sitting from lying manoeuvre shown in Figures 3.10 to 3.12 and described earlier is also very helpful in gaining control against gravity.

It is advisable to position the baby in prone position often during the day. This position will encourage movement of the head, resulting in an increase in the strength of the neck and back muscles. Many babies cannot push up on the elbows and

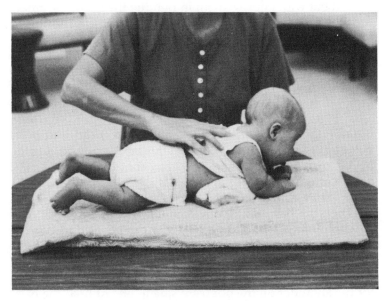

Figure 3.21 Using a towel for support under the chest.

benefit from the support of a rolled up small towel under the chest (Figure 3.21).

In making the roll, the edges of the towel should be turned in first so that the roll will have a depression in the middle for the chest while the bulk at the ends will give an extra lift to the shoulders. This position allows for movement of the head and provides good support through the arms. The baby's attention can be gained with the voice or with toys while the neck and back muscles are stroked with firm but gentle pressure from the pads of the fingers or the whole hand. If the baby has no head control, support can be given by placing a hand under the baby's chin. While stroking down the back, gradually raise the head just enough to give the baby the feel of the movement. To activate the muscles, the support can be reduced slightly thereby encouraging a stronger muscle contraction. As head control improves, the activities described previously can be introduced.

When the baby has enough head control to keep the head steady while held in a sitting position, the hands can be cupped around the baby shoulders and the baby swayed from side to side. Initially, a gentle swaying movement is used but with improvement in righting the head, the amplitude and speed of the sway can be increased until the opposite buttock lifts off the bed (or floor). After the movement to one side, the child should always be given time to respond.

ROLLING OVER

Usually the baby will not roll until some head and body postural control has been achieved but rolling may be initiated by a caregiver as soon as some head control is present. The baby's attention may be attracted by the voice or face of the carer, or by bright or musical toys.

When the baby is not developmentally ready to roll over independently, the following activity can be used to give the infant the 'feel' of the action. The hands are cupped over the baby's bent knees and the knees are moved from side to side. After each movement to one side, the caregiver should wait for the shoulder on the opposite side to lift. At first, the baby may not show this response and it may be necessary to stroke

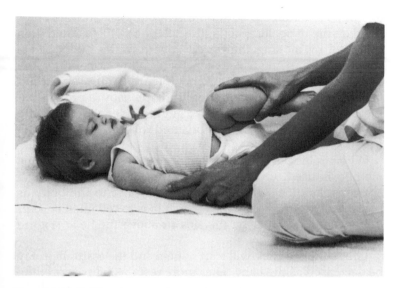

Figure 3.22 Rolling from supine to prone.

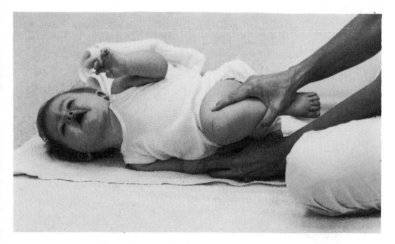

Figure 3.23 Continuing the roll.

or even gently lift that shoulder to give the child the feel of the movement.

When the baby starts to show an interest in rolling, this may be encouraged in the following way. With the baby in supine, one hand should be placed on the flexed knee and the other hand on the opposite arm (Figure 3.22). The child should then be rolled by moving the flexed knee towards the opposite shoulder. Care must be taken to tuck the arm under the body before removing the hand (Figure 3.23). The rolling movement should be continued until the baby is prone. If at the end of the roll, the arm is caught under the chest, the shoulder on that side should be lifted to allow the arm to be free.

When rolling the baby from prone to supine, the same method is used. One knee is bent and flexed towards the opposite shoulder while being kept as close to the body as possible. The arm over which the child is to roll must be kept fully extended, either by the side or above the head (Figure 3.24).

Gradually the baby will start to help and the assistance may be decreased as the baby takes more responsibility for rolling over. Less and less assistance will be required until a slight pull across the abdominals may be enough to initiate the movement. Once the baby has an idea of the movement, a toy can be placed out of reach to encourage the roll.

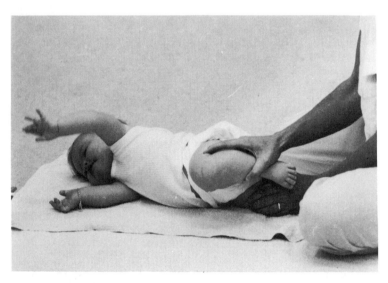

Figure 3.24 Rolling from prone to supine.

NOTE

One major aim of these activities is to encourage babies with Down syndrome to become responsible for their own movements rather than to rely passively on the actions of others. The need for enjoyable and motivating interactions should be paramount and care must be taken not to turn the activities into serious and possibly stressful teaching sessions. If the caregiver talks or sings to the baby while giving the movement practice, the activities will seem more like fun and will also expose the baby to the sounds and rhythms of speech.

4

Activities during the pre-toddler and toddler period

Rose-Anne Kelso and Sue Price

INTRODUCTION

During the pre-toddler and toddler period, there will be further development of the child's postural, locomotor, and manipulative skills. The quality of the toddler's actions will depend on the quality of the skills already acquired and on practice of desired patterns of movement. There are many movement activities to provide this practice that a physiotherapist can introduce to the caregiver and child with Down syndrome. Again, the most useful activities are those that can be adapted to become part of the normal day-to-day interactions between caregiver and child. Now that the child is older, the common daily routines of feeding, changing, bathing, and dressing offer even more opportunities for playful interactions and for practice of the desired movements.

FEEDING

Independent feeding needs to be encouraged despite the inevitable mess. It should be remembered that food is not only of nutritional value but it provides an avenue for tactile and fine motor experiences. Finger foods such as small cubes of food, sultanas and dried fruit are very useful at this stage. A small soft plastic medicine cup can be useful for introducing small quantities of liquid. Later, drinking from a beaker can be introduced. If the beaker has a flared rim (i.e. is bell-shaped), it is held so that the rim rests on the child's bottom lip and the tongue is kept inside the mouth. The flared rim helps the flow of liquid to be regulated allowing time for the child to gain control of lip and tongue action.

If the child is given tools for feeding, these should be suitable for grasping, light in weight, and designed for easy location of the food. By the time the child is ready to drink independently from a cup it is best to use one made of firm plastic with one or two handles. Children should be encouraged to hold their own cups while drinking. A cup with a straw may be helpful as it aids good tongue placement, lip closure, and general oral muscle control.

SITTING

Initially, when the child is placed in a sitting position, it is with the trunk supported. Independent sitting should be encouraged by gradually removing support from the trunk. As postural control and balance improve, the sitting position is more easily maintained and eye-hand co-ordination and manipulative abilities can be developed further. The child with good postural or equilibrium reactions is able to adopt various sitting postures and maintain them easily.

It should be noted that sitting is not a static state and that limb and trunk movements are to be encouraged while the child is in a sitting position. It should also be noted that once the motor skill of sitting is achieved, the tendency to always place the child in that position should be avoided. The essential feature of motor development is not the attainment of a motor milestone (e.g. sitting) but how it is incorporated into the overall development of motor function and skill.

Certain sitting positions, if used to the exclusion of all others, are not good for the child. One example is the child who sits 'between the knees' ('W' sitting, as in Figure 4.1). The internal rotation at the hip puts unnatural stress on the hip and knee joints.

Other positions which can inhibit progress include sitting forward between the hips (Figure 4.2) or sitting with the legs crossed (tailor sitting).

In these positions, the child can become 'stuck' and opportunities to practice balancing and changing positions are

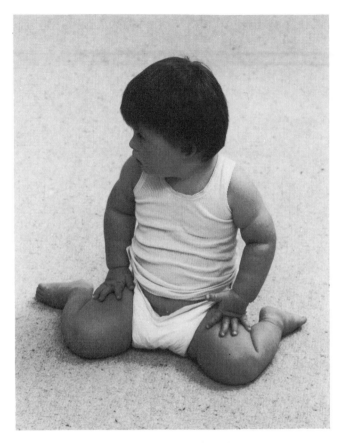

Figure 4.1 Do *not* allow the child to sit like this.

limited. The child in Figure 4.3 is sitting well and has much opportunity to move.

If children are sitting with their legs extended, it is important to make sure that they are sitting right back on their bottoms with the flexion occurring at the hips and not in the lower back. Sitting in the bath on a non-slip mat can provide enjoyable opportunities for practising a good sitting position.

As the child progresses and trunk muscles become stronger, sitting with the legs together or to one side are more

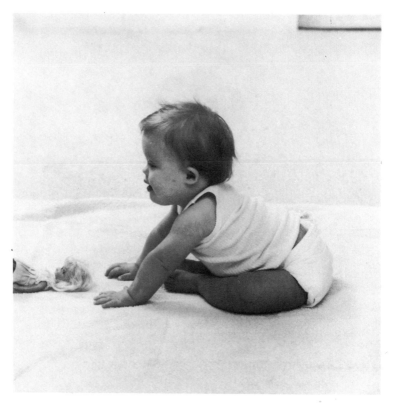

Figure 4.2 Do *not* encourage this sitting position.

demanding positions as they encourage trunk rotation and further balance and postural control (Figure 4.4). In this position, it is impossible to sit between the hips. The trunk rotation encouraged by side sitting also allows the child to move more easily on to hands and knees, thence to crawl or to stand up.

Due to the shortness of the arms, if the children require arm support for stability in sitting, it may be helpful to place their hands on their thighs but progression to more dynamic positions should be encouraged.

To maintain sitting during a variety of daily activities (bathing, eating, dressing and playing), protective and equilibrium

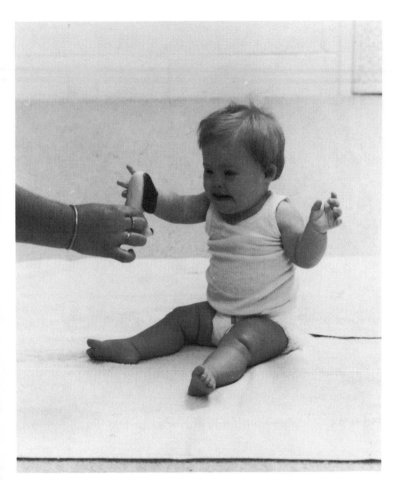

Figure 4.3 This child is sitting well.

reactions are required. The protective reactions of the arms in sitting form part of the balance mechanism. To assist in the initial development of these reactions, the child may need to be given the feeling of taking weight through the arms. This is done with the child in a sitting position. The therapist or caregiver should put one of the child's arms out to the side and firmly push down through it, keeping the

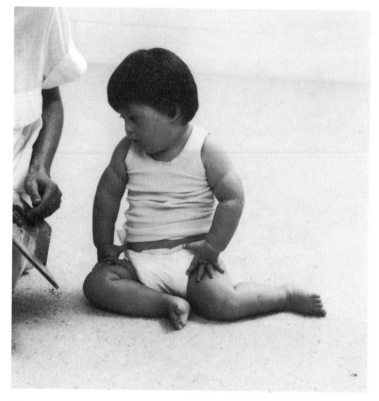

Figure 4.4 Side sitting when trunk muscles are stronger.

child's elbow straight by holding it with a hand (see Figure 4.5). Because children with Down syndrome often have relatively short limbs, it may be necessary to put a folded towel (or something similar) on either side of the child to allow the use of protective reactions. Once the child has the idea of these reactions, there may be no further need of the towel.

After this preparatory activity, the child can be gently tipped off balance to facilitate these rections automatically. Soon the child will use the protective reactions naturally during changes in position. This can be encouraged by placing toys to the side just out of reach.

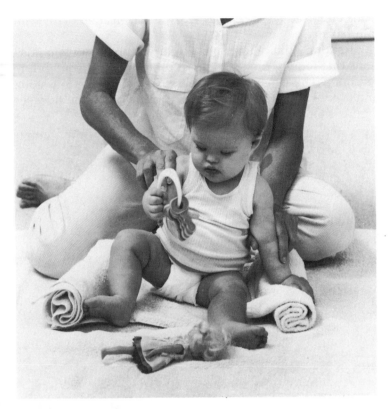

Figure 4.5 Taking weight through the arms.

Balance in sitting

The equilibrium reactions can be elicited by tipping the child off balance. Initially, the child will only be able to respond slowly but as children become more adept, they can be tipped more quickly. It must be remembered that persons of any age, if tipped off balance too quickly or strongly, will use their protective reactions.

At first, the child should be supported around the hips while being tipped. Once this can be managed, the child can be held round the knees and tipped in any position. When tipped to one side the child will bring the head and trunk to the midline and when tipped diagonally backwards, the trunk and head will be brought forward in an attempt to maintain balance.

As sitting balance improves, children can be put into positions that require the use of both protective and equilibrium reactions. This can be done by sitting the child on a low stool, and encouraging the child to reach up and out to the side (see Figure 4.6). This elicits good trunk rotation.

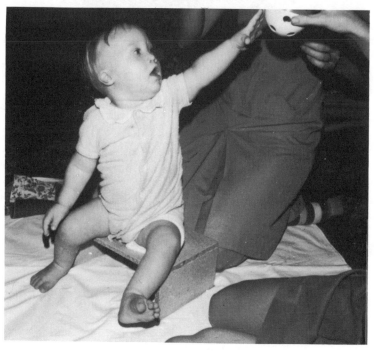

Figure 4.6 Eliciting trunk rotation.

PREPARATION FOR CRAWLING

There is some controversy about the need for, and the role of crawling. Crawling plays an important role in the development of muscle control round the hips and shoulders. If the fundamental experiences usually gained during crawling (rotation, weight shift, co-ordination and muscle control) are achieved in another way during development, the act of crawling itself need not be so important.

Good strength and tone in the hip, abdomen, back extensor and shoulder muscles and an ability to shift weight in all directions are essential components of four-point reciprocal crawling. Therapists should watch for hyperextension of the elbows as this will prevent muscular control round this joint. It is also important to make sure that the knees are under the hips and not widely abducted. Poor scapular stability and/or weak abdominals may be present and require attention. In order to develop control of these components, the following activities are appropriate.

With the therapist sitting on the floor and the child prone over the therapist's extended legs, the child can be positioned and encouraged to rock backwards and forwards. During this activity, the therapist is able to give proprioceptive input by pressing gently downwards through the child's bottom (Figure 4.7).

In the same manner, pressure can be applied through the child's shoulders when the child's arms are extended. The therapist should watch to see that the child takes the weight through the heel of the hand. The fingers will normally remain slightly flexed.

Alternatively, if the therapists legs are rolled, the child's weight will be moved backwards and forwards thereby

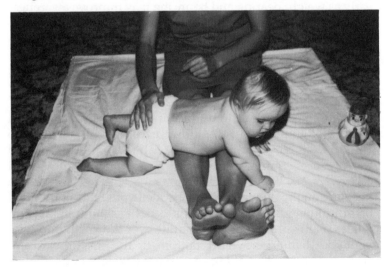

Figure 4.7 Preparation for crawling.

enabling weight and pressure to be taken through either the arms or legs in an alternating pattern.

Another activity which will encourage weight through the arms and help improve the strength and tone of the trunk muscles is one in which the child is held above a low table, taking weight through the arms. One of the therapist's hands supports the child's chest and the other holds the legs to ensure a good safe position.

As the strength in the arms increases, the support is decreased. This can be achieved by moving the support back to the hips and finally the legs. Walking along on hands and playing wheelbrrows, can then be tried with the child.

To encourage stability and to allow the feeling of self support, the child can be rocked gently backwards and forwards or from side to side while in the unsupported crawling position. Babies will often do this themselves before attempting to crawl alone. When ready, the child will crawl but an attractive object nearby may provide encouragement.

PREPARATION FOR STANDING AND WALKING

As the child attains independent sitting, pulling to stand can be encouraged. Supported standing can be introduced quite early as weight bearing and bouncing may improve awareness and control of the lower limbs. It is suggested that this builds up supportive reactions and develops muscle control. It is important for the child to take the weight on the soles of the feet. For a short period, some children may go through a period of not wanting to stand and either fail to extend the knees or actually bend both the hips and the knees.

Children often need to be encouraged to stand but should be allowed to proceed at their own pace. In order to develop a good basis for walking, plenty of time should be allowed for practice. Some practice activities for therapists and caregivers are illustrated in Figures 4.8 to 4.10. First, while kneeling on the floor and sitting back on your feet, sit the child on your knees so that the child's knees and hips are at right angles (Figure 4.8). Cup your hands over the knees and with your body behind the child's bottom, tip the hips forward and stand the child up, making sure that the weight ends up well forward over the child's feet (Figure 4.9 and Figure 4.10).

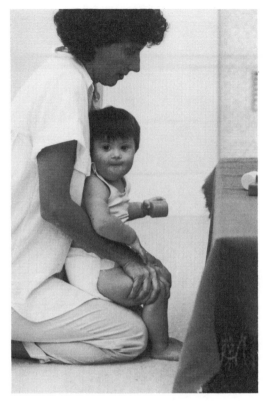

Figure 4.8 Encouraging the child to stand.

While in the standing position, help the child to feel weight by giving some pressure down through the legs. Doing these activities near a low table, will give the child a surface at a good height for playing. The support will also provide a little thoracic stability for safety and security.

Another way to aid standing is to place only one hand over the child's knees, the other one behind the bottom, and to then move the child's weight forward thus facilitating standing.

In order to encourage children to pull to stand by themselves, sit the child near a low, stable chair or coffee table that is suitable to hold for support. A desirable toy may be

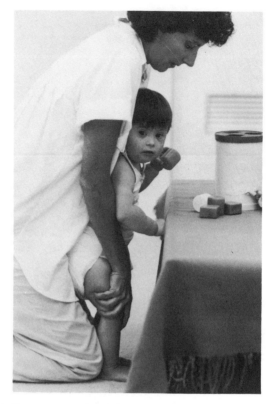

Figure 4.9 Encouraging the child to stand.

placed on the chair (or table) in such a way that standing is the only way of reaching it. The sequence is illustrated in Figures 4.11 to 4.13. Once the child is standing, activities involving weight transfer sideways and forwards can be initiated by using the hip as a key point. Weight transfer is an important component in walking and thus in motor development. Later, the child can be encouraged to cruise or traverse small gaps between stable supports.

Side stepping

The ability to take weight on only one leg is an essential

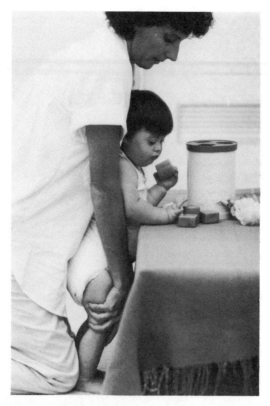

Figure 4.10 Encouraging the child to stand.

prerequisite for walking. The child should be placed near a stable support of appropriate height. Once the child is standing, the knee can be bent and the weight shifted on to the other leg (Figure 4.14). This position should be held for a few seconds to give the child the feel of the movement. The leg can then be let go so that it returns to the original position (Figure 4.15). If the child cannot maintain extension in the supporting (standing) leg, then keep the hip of the flexing leg in a neutral or extended (not flexed) position during this activity.

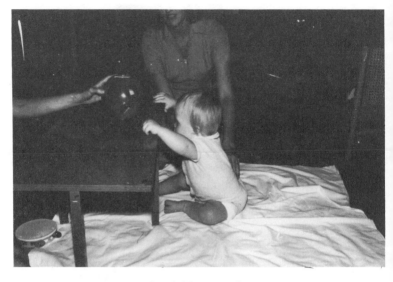

Figure 4.11 Encouraging the child to stand.

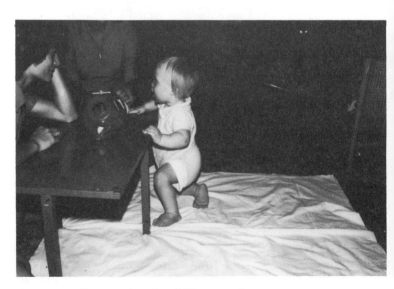

Figure 4.12 Encouraging the child to stand.

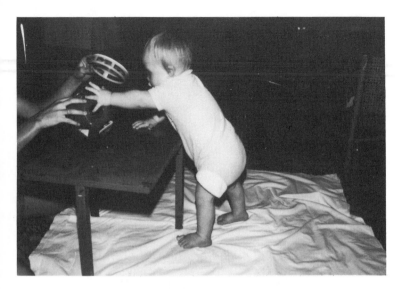

Figure 4.13 Encouraging the child to stand.

The same effect can be gained by gently tipping the child from the shoulder. This should always be done gently and the child given time to respond. In Figure 4.16, the previous activity is performed incorrectly. It may be observed that there is no correct weight shift to the left and no control or alignment of the hip.

To introduce cruising or side stepping, the child can be encouraged to take a side step by bending the right leg (as in Figure 4.14), then placing it down a few centimetres closer to the left leg. This will often cause the child to shift the left leg further to the left in an attempt to regain the initial, more comfortable base. Encouragement and practice of weight shift, stepping, trunk rotation and balancing will assist the child to gain confidence and enjoy attempting new adventures.

Some children need to be encouraged to move across small gaps and also to reach from one height to another (Figure 4.17).

Independent walking opens up a range of new and exciting opportunities but it is not an easy stage to achieve. Walking

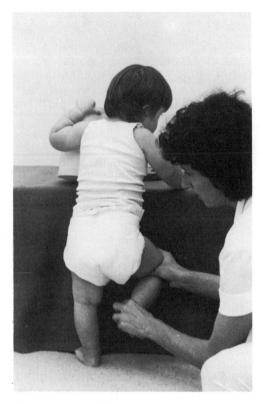

Figure 4.14 Helping the child to transfer weight.

involves co-ordination and an interplay of a large number of functions and reactions. These include postural and equilibrium reactions, muscle strength, control of muscle tone and integration of sensory input and feedback. Stepping out without support will occur when all is ready and the child is motivated to take the initiative. The long awaited first stage usually looks more like a waddle than a walk because the base is wide, the sideways weight shift is often exaggerated, the hips and knees are slightly bent and the arms held in abduction.

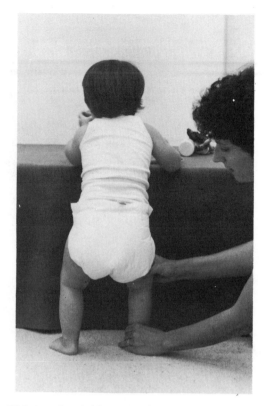

Figure 4.15 Helping the child to transfer weight.

Walking forward

To assist in the development of necessary control, a weighted object or small stable trolley may be useful to help improve forward walking (Figure 4.18). The caregiver's hands may be used to support walking but the amount of support should be gradually reduced and children should be encouraged to find their own centre of control.

To improve postural extension and awareness of the centre of gravity, the child may be stood with the back to a wall for support. Games such as 'clap hands' or 'give and take' may be useful in encouraging the child to stand with less

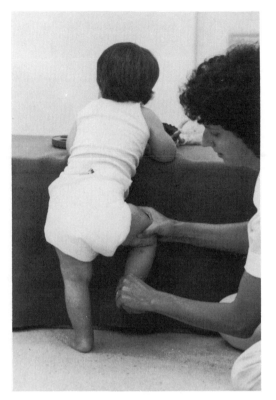

Figure 4.16 Incorrect alignment of hip, weight not transferred.

support from the wall. Once this has been achieved, the caregiver can move a short distance away so that the child has to take a few steps to reach either the caregiver or a desired object. Soon, independent steps will follow and often the child will soon progress to carrying an object while walking.

CLIMBING DOWN

Children love to climb but coming down can be difficult or even dangerous. Some learn to do this themselves but others

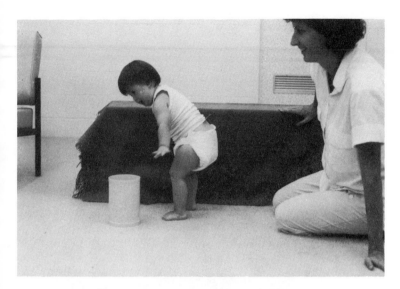

Figure 4.17 Side stepping.

need to be taught. There are many varied ways of doing it. The child, even with teaching, will use the easiest and most comfortable pattern but it is essential to make sure that it is a safe method.

The safest way to teach a child to get down off a bed or chair is shown from the starting position in Figure 4.19 to the final position in Figure 4.23. In the starting position, one leg is bent up and the body rotated (Figure 4.20). Rotation is continued over the leg by resting the trunk on the supporting surface. The child is on the tummy (Figure 4.21). The leg is then lifted out from under the body (Figure 4.22) and finally the child will slide down the front of the supporting surface to stand on the floor (Figure 4.23).

Stairs offer a similar challenge and the series of figures from Figure 4.24 to Figure 4.28 shows a good, safe way to descend stairs. A little at a time and performed slowly are the keys to success.

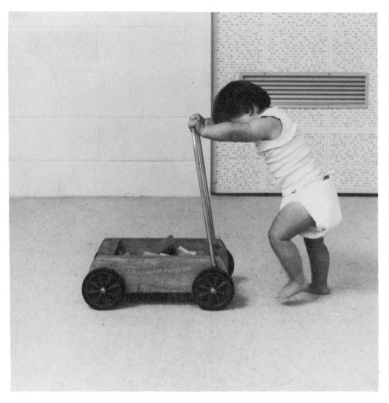

Figure 4.18 Trolley to help walking forward.

INCREASING AWARENESS

It is important in the early years to continue to give the child
stimulation to increase awareness of the body and its environment. The mobile, cruising or walking child can benefit from
sensory motor input. This can take the form of rough and
tumble play, rolling over and over down a slope or on a mat,
or spinning. Care should be taken to avoid exaggerated stretching of the muscles and joints or sudden movement of the
neck.

Circling round and round to increase input to the vestibular
system can be carried out with the child held or strapped in
a chair or swing. Start with two or three slow turns (about

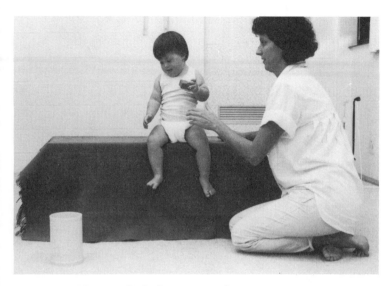

Figure 4.19 How to climb down: stage 1.

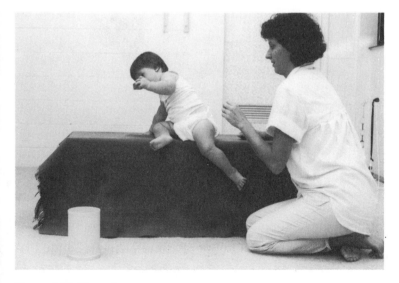

Figure 4.20 Stage 2.

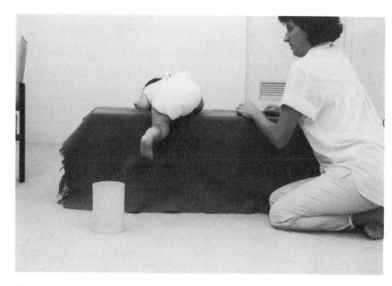

Figure 4.21 Stage 3.

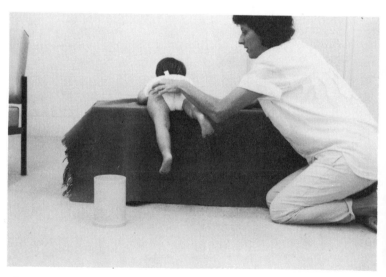

Figure 4.22 Stage 4.

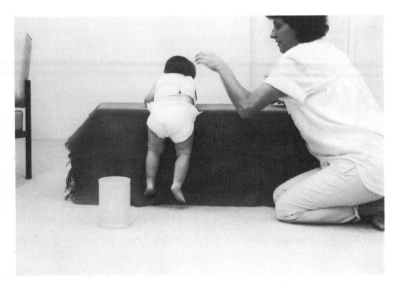

Figure 4.23 Stage 5.

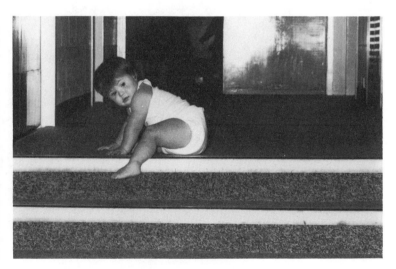

Figure 4.24 How to descend stairs: stage 1.

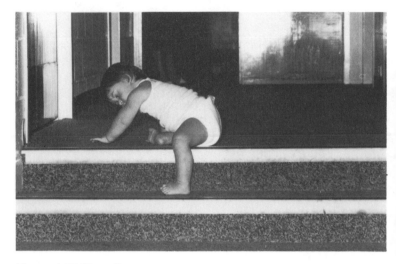

Figure 4.25 Stage 2.

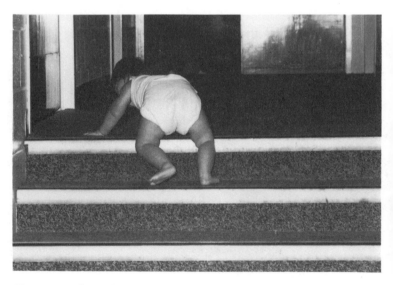

Figure 4.26 Stage 3.

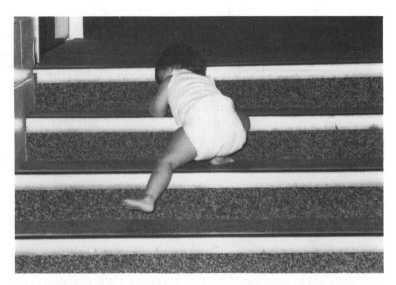

Figure 4.27 Stage 4.

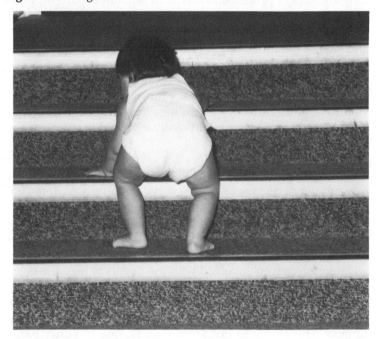

Figure 4.28 Stage 5.

one to two seconds per turn) in one direction followed by a rest of about 30 seconds, then repeat in the opposite direction.

Other activities include sitting the child (or placing the child on hands and knees) on a trampoline or similar surface then gently and rhythmically bouncing the surface while the child maintains the position. Introducing and playing with different textures and on various surfaces can provide experience with a variety of sensations. Bathtime provides another great opportunity. Games with a ball or a freely moving toy will encourage eye-hand co-ordination while rolling a bell or musical ball behind a screen may encourage movement with listening.

FINE MOTOR ACTIVITIES

Whereas babies develop their skills in reaching toward objects and grasping them, the older infant and toddler will develop greater skill in manipulating an object once it is grasped. The development of prehension follows a sequential pattern. From an early 'total hand' and palmar grasp, a more finite radial then pincer grasp develops. Pincer grasp between the thumb and side of the index finger gradually moves to the tips of the fingers.

Fine motor control is dependent on a number of factors other than the movement itself. Muscle tone and strength, postural stabilty, and sensory awareness provide an essential background for movement but motivation and practice are also very important.

Different motor experiences are very useful in helping the child to gain good hand control. Sophisticated and expensive toys are not necessary as many everyday household items will be just as varied and interesting.

The child may spend a lot of time transferring objects from one hand to the other and back again. Palmar grasp of the slightly bigger objects will improve (Figure 4.29). The thumb will become actively involved with the fingers to hold the object next to the palm.

Shortly after, the palm won't be needed so much for stabilization, and objects will tend to be held more in the fingers. The ability to hold two objects, one in either hand, tends to follow soon after.

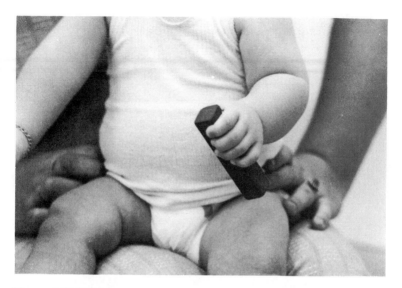

Figure 4.29 Palmar grasp.

There tends to be a surge of interest in toys about the stage when the baby can sit with hands free, crawl, and pull to stand. The child will often sit for some time placing objects in or under others and is perhaps developing a sense of the permanence of objects at this time. Plastic clothes pegs and kitchen containers are useful toys for this type of play.

Pointing (and poking) with the index finger becomes common, first as a means of exploring the properties of objects and later as a means of communication. Pointing allows the pre-verbal child to request or to express an interest in an object or activity to another person. Because that person often responds with the name of the object or a description of the activity, the acquisition of directed pointing is an important stage in the child's development of communication.

Increasing fine motor proficiencies can be seen also in activities such as tearing paper and 'posting' objects into small slots. The development of control of the intrinsic muscles of the hand will be evident in activities such as pulling toys by a string, scribbling, playing with blocks or using a spoon for eating and turning the pages of a book.

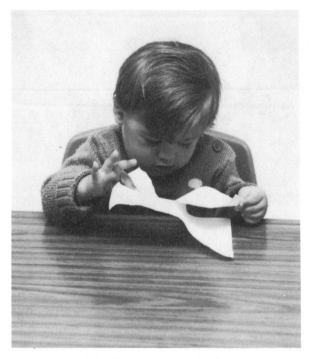

Figure 4.30 Fine motor proficiency.

WHAT HAPPENS NEXT?

Over the next few years, further movement skills will be developed as the child learns to walk confidently on different surfaces, to walk downstairs like an adult alternating each foot to a stair, to run and jump, to dance, to throw and catch a ball, to build with blocks, and to paint or draw a picture. The continuing development of these locomotor and manipulative skills allows more intensive exploration. This will lead to new skills and a greater appreciation of space, objects, and other people.

The preschool years will also provide the opportunity of learning from peers as the child learns to work and play in a group. The toddler may be eager to play but has not yet learnt the skills of helping, sharing and taking turns. The busy preschooler learns many of these complex social skills and interactions with other children will become an important part of the child's life.

5

The active preschooler

Louise Mercer

Remarkable changes in development take place during the preschool years. This has been well described by Laszlo and Bairstow (1985), 'There is a process of progressively building on what has already been established, a development of knowledge of relationships between sensory and motor events within and across time, and a progressive differentiation and accretion of knowledge that is achieved through action, and this knowledge in turn modifies behaviour.' (p. 43).

Exploration of the immediate environment occurs through the senses of vision, hearing, touch, movement, and tasting. Deprivation of stimuli to any of these senses may inhibit the development of that sense, and distort the processing of more complex stimuli in the future. Many children with Down syndrome have clinically recognizable problems with vision, hearing or oro-motor dysfunction. Due to differences in the structure of the tongue and mouth and difficulties in co-ordinating rapid movement, the ability to discover texture, taste, and form of objects or food may be restricted. There may be poor quality movement because of the low tone of the muscles, poor general health, perhaps congenital heart problems, and repeated upper respiratory infections. Any one of these problems can affect the processing of the stimuli required for normal sensori-motor development.

Many writers testify to the importance of appropriate sensory development in the acquisition of normal motor development (Twitchell, 1954; Clark *et al.*, 1977; Goodkin, 1980; Laszlo and Bairstow, 1985). With a poor background of developing sensory awareness it is understandable that children with Down syndrome can appear as clumsy, poorly co-ordinated preschoolers with motor skills below the level of their peers.

How can this problem be addressed? Sensory and motor development is multi-faceted, and for a young child it needs to be part of play. Any additional or special stimulation needs to be goal-oriented, so that the activities have meaning for the children and caregivers. Activities need to be easily repeated at home so that repetition and positive reinforcement of the stimuli can promote integration within the child's repertoire of skills. To promote a motor response, there should be visible outcomes from the child's reaction to the stimulation and it needs to be fun!

There are often a number of different people with different specialized skills who are in contact with the child with Down syndrome and the family. Combining these people into a team and bringing them together with the caregivers and children is an efficient way of helping the families. Team members involved with children with special needs include caregivers, therapists (physiotherapists, occupational therapists, speech therapists), and teachers (often specialized in skills of special education or early childhood and development).

A playgroup forms an ideal setting where caregivers and children have the opportunity to meet with peers as well as to interact with a variety of team members. It is a setting where a transdisciplinary team functions appropriately. Regular involvement of the team allows for flow of information and cross-skilling of the team members. In the relaxed setting of the playgroup, caregivers and children are spared the stress of appointment times and the time-induced pressures to perform. Not only do the caregivers and children learn through both structured and unstructured experiences but the teachers and therapists are more likely to observe the usual dynamics of caregiver-child interactions. The benefits for the child of working within a group are enhanced. Competition amongst peers provides natural challenges while encouragement from peers nurtures group membership and opportunities for helping and sharing.

Each of the professionals in the team can observe the children and what they do as they play and interact with their environment. Individual assessment by each of these professionals and sharing of these assessments amongst the team members can provide a valuable profile of each child's abilities. Areas of dysfunction can be identified and prioritized. Specific goals can be set for each child and methods of achieving these goals planned and built into playgroup and home activities.

This process of assessment, sharing knowledge, setting goals and planning provides the basis for efficient and effective programming. Transdisciplinary teams must allocate sufficient time for adequate assessment and planning if the period that children spend at the playgroup is to be of specific benefit to each child. It is important to see the children in the group in terms of their individual needs.

Based on the information gained from individual assessments, the physiotherapy aims incorporated into playgroups may be summarized as the following:

1. to facilitate improved motor performance by neuro-sensory stimulation of input systems;
2. to develop the musculoskeletal abilities, keeping in mind the anatomical structure and alignment of the body;
3. to stimulate perceptual-motor skills;
4. to introduce opportunities for generalization of skills;
5. to develop effective communication skills;
6. to improve exercise tolerance while being aware of possible physical limits.

A knowledge of child development can give a background for the playgroup's activities. Whereas a three year old will often enjoy cutting and glueing, a two year old will find it difficult and tedious. Children of all ages, however, may enjoy sand and water play. In a multi-aged group, a teacher with early childhood experience can plan the use of suitable activities through which motor skills are practised while maintaining the interest and motivation of the children.

Children often play on the floor. The posture and abilities a child exhibits when playing on the floor can give the therapist insight into the functional level of that child. Children who have head and trunk control can sit independently with arms free to move while the development of hand-eye co-ordination then enables the introduction of tools, be they rattles, eating utensils, pencils, or computer keyboards. Usually the achievement of sitting from supine (lying on the back) requires the abilities of rolling, prone propping, pulling up into four point kneeling, swivelling into side-sitting, and righting oneself from a stretched side-sitting posture to a balanced erect trunk over a stable base. Long before infants can do this, it is common for them to be propped and positioned in a sitting position. Having experienced this sitting position, children often then seek to acquire that position so that they can view a more interesting environment.

Equipment (inflated rollers, bean bag chairs or rolls, stools or boxes) may be helpful in exposing the child to the position

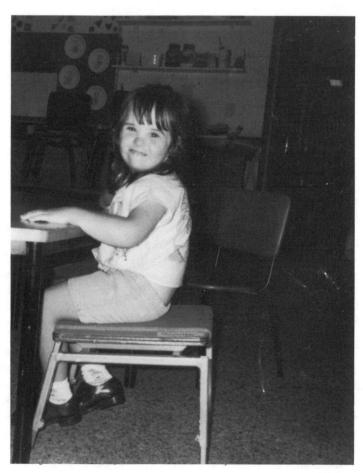

Figure 5.1 A tilt stool.

and posture of sitting but techniques to improve the segmental sequence required in attaining sitting are also necessary. An understanding of the movement sequences often used by children is valuable when helping the child who cannot achieve the sequence independently. Some ideas for providing this help have been presented in the previous chapter (Kelso and Price). Once the child can sit, the use of inflated inner tube rings, cushions, stools, padded toy boxes, or tilt stools can provide the child with a variety of experiences in sitting.

To allow freedom of hands for play and activity, a child needs to be stable, well aligned but posturally dynamic in sitting. Tilt stools can be very effective aids to the establishment of a stable well-aligned sitting posture (see Figure 5.1). Adjustments can be made to the leg height, front and back, in order to cater for leg length. The slope of the chair can be adjusted so that the weight-bearing anatomical surfaces can be altered.

For example, a child may be observed when sitting on the floor, to have an immature 'C' shaped spinal curve, the head may be tilted backwards, the jaw open, the tongue thrusting forwards, shoulders rounded, belly protruding, and legs positioned to give as wide a base as possible (either splayed into abduction, legs crossed, or internally rotated at the hips with knees bent in a 'W' shape). This child can be put on a tilt stool with the rear legs higher than the front so that the child's body weight is tipped forwards. The feet need to be flat on the floor to take the forwards inclination, the knees are brought closer together to transmit the body weight, a lumbar curve is seen in place of the rounded spine and the shoulders are back while the child may sometimes need to push down on the arms to maintain this erect trunk posture.

Providing action and activities in this position gives the child practice at maintaining this posture and a positive alternative to the child's previously preferred immature sitting style. The anti-gravity muscle groups which are enlisted to hold the posture will strengthen over time. The advantages of an erect but stable posture over a slouched immature posture need to be recognized and reinforced by all those interacting with the child. It is important also that the process of attaining sitting through the rolling, placing, and propping, then hitching into four point kneel and rotational weight shift through side sitting, to sitting on the floor in a controlled, upright fashion be practised.

Using the tilt stool whilst performing some other playgroup activity reinforces this erect, upright posture. Team members should be aware of the need for reinforcement of correct posture and either use some form of equipment, such as the tilt stool, to facilitate the appropriate posture or remind children to correct their positions during the ordinary daily activities as well as during directed play. Stability in sitting provides a base from which other skills may be developed e.g. visual attention, communication, whether verbally or by signing, upper limb mobility and dexterity, and the ability to interact with a variety of tactile media e.g. play-doh, paint, shaving-cream, clay or crayons.

To move from sitting to standing, that is, leaning forward, straightening the knees and taking weight through the feet, requires stability about the hips and pelvic girdle. A co-ordinated interplay of hip flexor, extensor, and abductor muscles is essential for this action. Abdominal muscle groups and trunk extensors are essential also to fix the position of the trunk so that the child does not overbalance as the weight is moved forward. A variety of automatic postural righting and equilibrium reactions must work together to ensure this does not happen. Balance of the body over the feet must be experienced and learnt, before movement from the standing position can be achieved. Standing with less and less support from in front and from behind, will assist the child to gain the necessary experience, control and confidence.

As explained in the previous chapter (Kelso and Price), pulling to stand and cruising (stepping sideways while holding on to a firm support) provide valuable preparation for walking. These activities not only strengthen the muscles of the lower limbs but promote control of weight shift in standing and require the child to achieve dynamic stability around the hips and pelvis.

In many children with Down syndrome, independence in walking will be delayed and an immature pattern will remain for some time. Assessing the quality of the gait is important for planning ways to improve it. This assessment should include evaluation of the width of the dynamic base, control of all joints of the lower limbs and pelvis, the method and distance of the step, the angle of foot placement, the ability to step forward with a narrower base (stride) and the pattern or rhythm of the overall gait cycle.

Some characteristics observed in children with Down syndrome include a persistence of a wide base, a lack of dynamic stability (compensated sometimes by over-fixation), an inability to step forward (central rotation) and a lack of rhythm and 'toe-off' in the cycle, resulting in a rather heavy movement.

Attainment of independent walking is eagerly sought and once achieved there can be a tendency to consider that there

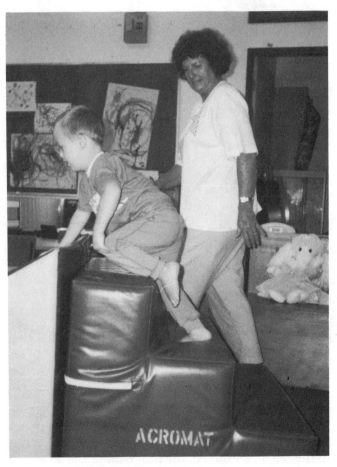

Figure 5.2 A climbing game.

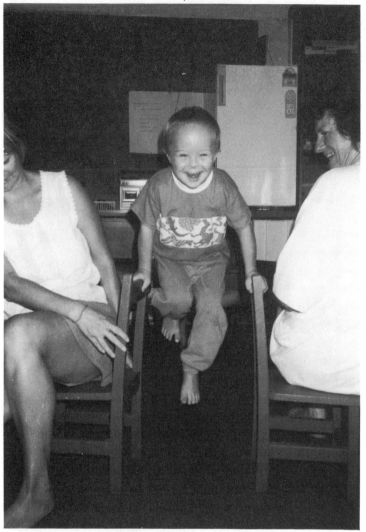

Figure 5.3 Another climbing game.

is nothing further for the physiotherapist to do. This is not the case because poor quality gait can have effects on the biomechanics of functional movement, placing undue stress on muscles and joints.

At this stage, one aim of the programme will be to improve dynamic stability around the lower trunk and hips particularly in positions which involve rotational patterns of movement. This may be accomplished during floor activities (sitting and crawling), standing (reaching, bending and squatting), and climbing games.

Climbing on to a chair, a ladder, a ride-on toy or an adult's back for a ride provide opportunities to practise controlled rotational movement patterns. Progression may include stepping over a rope on to a stepping stone or later, on to a step.

Sitting, kneeling or standing or a trampoline mat or similar surface will provide the opportunity to be put off balance,

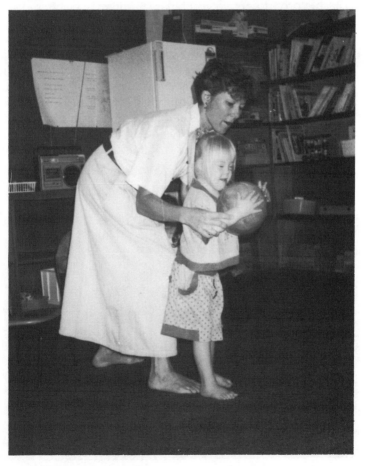

Figure 5.4 Learning to play.

facilitating the use of postural and equilibrium reactions while giving the opportunity to fall safely. Obstacle courses and resisted push-pull type activities can be used to strengthen muscle groups and improve automatic weight shift. To be able to provide a programme that encompasses all of these forms of stimulation within an acceptable amount of family time is a challenge but structuring the activities about play is an efficient way of meeting this challenge.

Some helpful themes to use include the following.

1. **Adventures with senses** This is a time when a variety of tactile/proprioceptive/vestibular stimuli may be offered e.g. vibration, stroking, paint brushing, playing with various media, rocking, jumping, rolling in blankets or sheets.
2. **Physio Frolics** This provides a chance for individual assessment of current needs, and the delivery of specific treatment techniques to meet these needs. It is important to relate directly to the family's perceived needs. Many of these relate to activities of daily living. Examples include sitting well while the child is being fed or self feeding is being introduced, use of rotational positions during

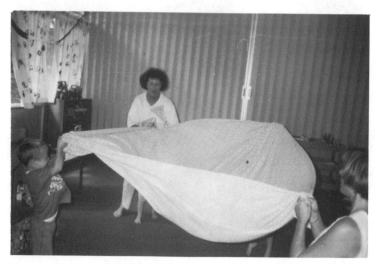

Figure 5.5 Adventures with senses.

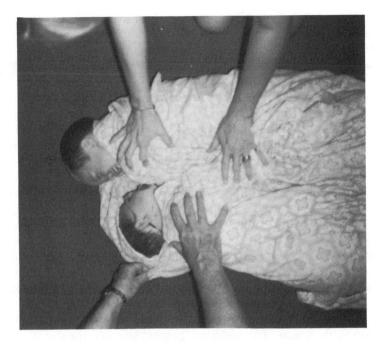

Figure 5.6 More adventures with senses.

dressing, and stimulation of neck and trunk to promote and maintain an erect sitting posture. Other activities during dressing include reaching with hands up to put arms into sleeves, standing on one leg while pants are changed, or balancing in sitting while shoes and socks are put on.

3. **Sitting with structure** This time is spent in sitting, be it on a parent's lap, an appropriate tilt stool, the floor, or a normal chair. The seated posture should have these main characteristics:
   (a) head midline
   (b) symmetrical shoulder joints
   (c) straight spine
   (d) symmetrical hips
   (e) feet flat on the floor or on a flat support.

Once a satisfactory posture is achieved the child must be given the opportunity to use it. Integrating visual and auditory attention to a source of stimulation whilst maintaining postural stability is a pre-requisite for many academic functions. There are a number of activities which can be used to combine sensory stimulation with a motor response. These can be lots of fun whether they involve ocular-motor or auditory-motor systems. Trying to catch bubbles or visually tracking a sparkler or torchlight or an animated toy that is being moved in front and across the body. High pitched bells tinkling, or the rat-tat-tat or ping-ping of a toy can arrest the attention of even the most passive and seemingly disinterested child.

The incentive to catch and play with these toys may be used to stimulate eye-hand co-ordination or improve the attention of a visually inattentive child. Respiratory skills of blowing, inhaling, puffing, or increasing the strength of a forced voluntary expiration can all be facilitated through the use of candles, streamers or mobiles. One candle encourages one puff and many candles require larger breath and force of expiration. A line of candles requires a breath/blow pattern that is also useful when a child is learning how to swim.

Follow the leader games can be used to mix sensory stimulation with action. The sensory 'games' suitable for the playgroup depend on the ages of the members. The following format is suggested for a group of three to six year olds and provides an example of sensori-motor FUN!

Adventures with ... The teacher may choose to introduce a new type of switch toy, the speech therapist may tell a story with signs and sounds, or the occupational therapist might have a session in food preparation where the children break eggs, noting the textures, the consistency and the force needed to do the breaking, and then each child in the group takes turns in adding milk, mixing, and lifting the mixture into the oven to cook.

At this time professional roles are not usually clearly delineated. In practice all the participants would be using language suitable for varying levels of communication, teachers would be helping in positioning for optimal stability on the chairs, the occupational therapist would be relating the 'academic' concepts of weight, measurement and number, while the physiotherapist and speech therapist may be facilitating a conversation and accompanying arm gestures from a child who had been asked about the whole procedure.

Picnic in the park provides another avenue for extending the child's sensori-motor experiences and abilities through activities such as picking up leaves, walking along a narrow beam, stepping on stones, throwing bread to the ducks, carrying the lunch bag, and playing bat the ball (with two hands on the handle to facilitate trunk rotation). Playground equipment such as tyre swings and climbing frames will often motivate a child to higher achievement.

Morning tea This can be an active intervention time where feeding and drinking habits may be observed and intervention offered, if necessary. It may be a more relaxing time when parents and professionals can discuss the outcomes of their playgroup's activities, the results of their intervention, its value or its shortcomings. As a regular forum on general progress, discussion over a cup of tea can be most informative. Of course regular reassessment and re-evaluation of goals and priorities are essential to maintain the individual orientation of the programme.

Music and movement Children with Down syndrome often show problems with head control, dissociation of eye movement from movement of the head position, problems with trunk stability and the automatic postural reactions of head and body righting, hypotonia, and hyper-extensible joints, poor co-contraction for stabilizing joints and weak anti-gravity muscle groups. Music provides an avenue for stimulating a variety of activities that will help in these problem areas. Nodding in time to the music, clapping to a rhythm, stamping feet, or kicking to the beat are simple movements made more meaningful when music is being played. Swinging scarves across the body, swirling them around in circles, or using instruments to bang, jiggle, press, scrape, or blow add complexity to simple stepping or marching to the music.

Music tapes with age-appropriate tunes can be designated as stabilizing songs, as fast action songs, or as fine motor songs. At the finish of a music session, the playgroup's session seems appropriately ended and this works well to let the children know that they too are finished for the day. The powerful aspect of repetition in learning a new skill is readily available through the use of music, with verse and chorus repeated in the song. Verbal cueing of a desired action is available in the words of well-known songs and movement, while rhythm and timing are encouraged through the music of simple songs.

The variety of formats for a playgroup is unlimited. Even for the same group of children, priorities of the individuals change, and so the nature of the playgroup must change to address these priorities.

There comes a time when the children will graduate from the rather informal playgroup to a more structured school programme. To help them achieve this transition successfully, activities are required that involve attending, following directions, and using a pencil or crayon.

In the more informal setting, activities such as playing with spring loaded pegs, paper tearing or collage, cooking, threading and fingerpainting are important in developing the strength, control and refinement of movement necessary for pencil activities. There are many skills involved in pencil use, however, and each child's readiness to draw or write with a pencil must be carefully monitored.

The variability in motor milestone and skill acquisition was noted in earlier chapters, and this variability in motor function continues through the lives of those with Down syndrome. The trandisciplinary team model with a focus on individualized activities is appropriate not only for children of preschool age but also for older groups that function with the aim of promoting good quality motor and physical skills. Regular exercise, joy in movement, satisfaction in the physical performance, social interaction and fun can be appreciated throughout the child's lifetime.

6

Play and movement education

Anne Jobling

Movement becomes a means through which children can express, explore, develop and interpret themselves and their relationships to the world in which they live.

Gallahue, Werner and Leudke, 1975 (p. 241)

INTRODUCTION

Play is a universal and dominant behaviour in childhood. It is pleasurable, spontaneous and positively valued. The feeling of enjoyment that children gain from play may be the primary motivating force but to remain enjoyable, a child's play experiences need to balance the abilities of the child with the challenges of the play.

Csikszentmihalyi (1975) has termed the condition occurring when there is a balance between skill and challenge as 'flow experience'. It is not a static condition, but allows for the provision of new stimuli and activities to engage attention and skill. According to Csikszentmihalyi, 'flow' is primarily concerned with the feelings generated from an activity and an important corollary is that if activities are sufficiently engaging to be practised and varied, the children both gain skills and enjoy themselves.

For many children with Down syndrome, practice and repetition are essential for the development of their repertoire of skills, and play is often used by therapists and teachers as a medium to provide these essential components. Adult sensitivity to the child's feelings may be needed, however, lest play which was at first fun, drifts into tedium and ceases to provide enjoyment to the child. It is also important that enjoyment not be lost as the early play experiences of preschoolers become more formalized in childhood games and sports.

In investigating the personal and situational factors prior to and immediately following a soccer game for 11–12 year old players, Scanlan and Passer (1981) reported that the level of 'fun' in the play was reflected in the players' overall satisfaction with the game experience. Fun was associated with the players' feelings of satisfaction with their own performance and the team's experience. Whether players won or lost, fun reduced the stress of the game. This finding has relevance for those structuring the play and games of children with Down syndrome as anxiety in games, especially in integrated settings, has been reported (Levine and Langness, 1983).

The play of children with Down syndrome is likely to differ from that of their normally developing peers. Early studies based on research with children in institutional settings reported that the children were passive interactors with their environment and were limited in their play initiatives. Their use of play space was reported to be more erratic as they moved more frequently and more slowly than other children (Linford *et al.*, 1971). The nature of their movement was described as continuous, and at a low activity level. Wade (1973) reported that their play appeared to have a flat and asocial perspective and according to Ellis and Scholtz (1978) 'it was as if these children did not possess the wherewithal to extract information from the setting and it was the featurelessness of their behaviour that became obtrusive leading to their isolation from society.' (p. 129).

Linford and Duthie (1970) concluded that, as the children could be encouraged to actively engage with the environment, the observed inactivity in free play was due to psychological/ behavioural problems rather than to physiological problems. One could not but wonder whether these children were bored in an institutional setting.

The more recent studies were no longer limited by their institutional nature but many were limited by small sample size (Li, 1981). Consequently, the results of the various studies were not always compatible with each other. Riguet and Taylor

(1981) reported that children with Down syndrome tended to be more repetitive in their play, constantly choosing familiar objects. McConkey (1985), however, thought it was difficult to define the precise nature of the play differences. He reviewed several studies of play and concluded that possible differences may be found in activity levels, exploratory ventures, and manipulation of objects.

Cunningham *et al.* (1984) and Beeghly *et al.* (1989) have suggested that the characteristics observed in the previous studies may have reflected delays in development and that a more fruitful approach might be to focus on the nature of the context in which the play interactions took place, for example, the physical environment (McConkey, 1980; Katz and Singh, 1986; Jones, 1987), mother-child interactions or therapist-child interactions (McConkey and Martin, 1983; McEnvoy and McConkey, 1983; Gunn and Berry, 1990) and play with peers (Ellis and Scholtz 1978, Guralnick and Groom 1985, 1988; Guralnick, 1990; Sloper *et al.*, 1989).

After observing the social context of play for preschoolers with Down syndrome, Sloper *et al.* (1990) concluded that they played more frequently with younger peers. These play arrangements were often organized by parents who continued to do this into later childhood. These researchers also indicated that the children with Down syndrome were less capable of structuring and organizing their play activity spontaneously. When using equipment they were significantly less creative and did not demonstrate variety and difference in their choices. It appeared that they may have needed help to play.

Many studies of play have been concerned with the relationship between play and cognitive or language skills, hence the notion that it may be worthwhile helping children to play. Moreover, references to the role of movement and physical skills have most often been made in a therapy context. Consequently, play tends to be seen as a 'serious business' for these children and fun seems to be ignored.

Yet the fun of moving and the participation in vigorous physical activity during play is very much part of the young child's world.

Movement is a prime element in young children's play and has a significant influence on their ability to participate in

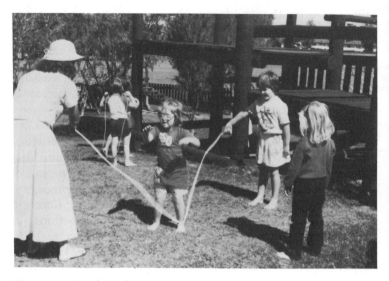

Figure 6.1 The fun of play.

formal and informal games. Yet research data on relationships between children's play, motor development and physical activity is sparse (Bergen, 1988).

Most studies of the early motor development of children with Down syndrome have described the acquisition of motor milestones (for example, Share and French, 1974). During the establishment of early intervention programmes for these children in the 1960s and 1970s, research was directed towards the development of curricula items and checklists for gross and fine motor development (Hayden and Haring, 1978; Pieterse *et al.*, 1988). The trampoline, scooter board, rope swings, puzzles and peg boards became popular pieces of equipment, and patterning, the physical manipulation of the body and the limbs to obtain movement, was often part of the physical programmes for these children. The sequence of the attainment of skills was emphasized but not the relationship between play and motor development.

The focus on skills for their own sake in early intervention programmes has given play a sombre nature. The over-zealous promotion of directed activities from checklists or 'recipe-type' developmental schemes or intensive training programmes has in some cases created situations where children refuse to play with toys and hide themselves under tables. Toys produced by therapists have been hidden under the carpet. As Sheridan (1977) was moved to remark 'some of the so-called play I have seen pressed upon handicapped children ... has been perilously close to drudgery.' (p. 13).

Different methods of intervention may be more effective than intensive training (Sloper *et al.*, 1986) and Cole (1986) has cautioned against the artificial nature of contrived settings for play interactions. Intervention programmes need to limit their adult control of play so that children with Down syndrome can experience the freedom of playful activity. There is value in stress-free play for children (Rokosz, 1987) and the maintenance of fun and enjoyment in intervention programmes has positive implications for practice and repetition of activities.

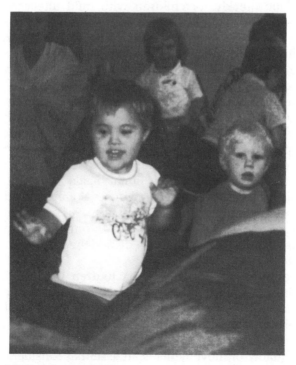

Figure 6.2 Joyful movement.

According to Brown (1980), 'children's lives are filled with spontaneous, joyful movement: they respond totally to their world with their heads, hearts and bodies.' (p. 282).

There is no reason why this should not apply for children with Down syndrome. Have we forgotten these aspects of play and the child's joy in our zeal to try to achieve cognitive gains?

FUNDAMENTAL MOTOR PATTERNS

The gross motor milestone of walking has often been regarded as the goal of intervention but other basic patterns of children's movements such as climbing and throwing need to be considered for their role in developing play skills. If children's movement abilities are poor, slow or deficient, then much time and energy in play may be directed towards moving rather than to the play activity or the game itself. Titus and Watkinson (1987) reported that play in integrated settings often moved too quickly for children with mild intellectual disabilities. As a result the children were unable to sustain contact and gave up trying to take part. It may be expected then that a lack of competence in moving and in understanding the game will handicap children with Down syndrome in fast-paced environments such as a playground.

Moreover, the resulting confusion and despondency at being unable to take part in the play may mean that they fall further and further behind others, not only in motor skill development but also in social skills. Substantial deficits in group play and child-child interactions as well as a lack of progression in social interactional skills with increased chronological age have been noted in developmentally delayed preschoolers (Guralnick and Weinhouse, 1984). Acquiring skill is difficult enough without these additional handicaps. The final result is that the children are denied the enjoyable aspects of physical play.

Holle (1976) suggested that if children with intellectual disabilities were to deal with both understanding the movements of the game and performing its skills, small group practice of movement patterns and skills were required as well as careful illustrations of the nature of the game.

The quality of movements is an essential consideration in the sequential development and acquisition of fundamental motor patterns and skills. We need to be interested in how the child with Down syndrome moves and plays. Efficient and effective movement prevents injury and encourages an ongoing positive attitude to activity.

Fundamental motor patterns and skills are regarded as the dynamic building blocks of more specific skills developed later in childhood. They may be considered as a continuum of regular and observable sequences of change in the way that children use their bodies to perform a particular movement e.g. running, skipping, throwing, and striking (Seefeldt and Haubenstricker, 1982; Wickstrom, 1983; Gallahue, 1989). The mature pattern provides a foundation for the development of game and sport skills. For example, throwing skill provides a foundation for a netball pass, a tennis serve and a baseball pitch. Knowledge of the levels of difficulty in skills such as skipping and jumping and an understanding of the sequence of development, assists the observer to individualize the movement experiences. The qualitative aspects of these sequences or patterns of movement involve and reflect the smoothness, timing, range and body's involvement in the movement.

Children with immature motor patterns may lack not only a sound basis for skill development, but also an adequate movement-knowledge base to make the feedback from moving relevant and meaningful. One can often observe that these children become overwhelmed by 'movement' information. They lose concentration and also the motivation to continue practising or persisting with the movement. This awareness of the movement experience is important and has significance for physical activities and games such as those which involve balance in hopping, jumping and striking. For skill acquisition, such feedback information from the movement is relevant and meaningful. Without such awareness, the learner of a skill can be inundated with all the information provided by the body and by the teacher. This then impacts on the long term development of patterns and skills. This may be especially true of the learner with an intellectual disability (Horgan, 1980; Sim and Stewart, 1984). It is important to remember nevertheless that for all children, whether they have Down syndrome or not, there are inconsistencies and loss of concentration in performance during childhood years. If such behaviours are shown, they should not be automatically attributed to the syndrome.

Several studies have examined the fundamental skills and patterns of children with intellectual disabilities. Ryan (1977) and Hemmert (1979) used the Ohio State University Scale of Intra Gross Motor Assessment and indicated that there is a delay in reaching the mature level of a skill. They suggested that qualitative differences in the skills existed in comparison with normally developing children. Climbing patterns were a particular focus in the Hemmert study (1979), and the observations and the measurements demonstrated that boys and girls with moderate retardation (C.A. 9–15 years) achieved a mature level (Level 4) by C.A. 12–15 years in comparison with non-handicapped children who achieved this level at six years of age (Ryan 1977). Loovis (1989) examined the environmental factors in the development of climbing and stressed the necessity to focus on climbing activities and equipment that matched the proficiency level of the children and the adults with intellectual disabilities. In particular, the circumference of the rungs is important for children with Down syndrome whose hand and foot sizes tend to be smaller and shorter. Loovis stressed that for both adults and children, it is important to develop a mature climbing pattern with appropriate equipment before providing experiences in a community recreational setting.

Holland (1987) examined seven fundamental motor skills of children aged from six to ten years who were described as educationally mentally retarded. He found that although the children were slower in acquiring a mature pattern, the normal developmental sequences of the skill could be observed. The children showed improvement over time (with differences in favour of the males) on throw, bounce, kick and strike performances. Improvements were attributed to environmental factors such as practice and the nature of available opportunities.

There may be a regression in motor skill patterns as children with intellectual disabilities grow older because of decreased maturity in gait patterns and a less active lifestyle (Wickstrom, 1983). Poor motor abilities may be due more to such factors than to the level of cognitive functioning. Holle (1976) believed that the poor performance and fitness of older children

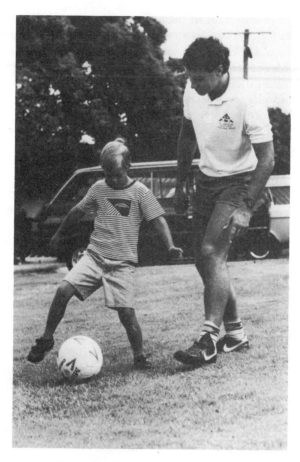

Figure 6.3 Trying for a goal (Reproduced with permission of *The Courier-Mail* of Brisbane, Australia.).

with intellectual disabilities could be attributed partly to late development and partly to lack of movement opportunities, but suggested that they could be improved through daily activities.

Walking

Walking is the milestone most eagerly awaited by parents and many early stimulation programmes focus on this task. It is important, however, to analyse and monitor the performance of this new skill and not to only note that the milestone has been achieved. *How* the task is performed is an important factor for lifelong efficiency of the skill. Walking is a form of locomotion and has two phases, the swing and the support phases, which require leg strength for support, and maintenance of stability to transfer weight. Children with Down syndrome often exhibit a wider than normal base of support in walking and experience some foot angle problems especially intoeing (Parker and Bronks, 1980). In the support phase, five year olds lack a certain level of stability which produces an inability to achieve normal step length and also an increased flexion at the hip and knee joint in order to maintain balance (Parker *et al.*, 1986). Some also exhibit diminished control of the ankle joint.

General movement activities that focus on awareness of the body parts involved (head, trunk, knees, feet and arms) as well as the development of overall strength, control and balance can help improve the gait. Shoes should be chosen so that they provide good support to prevent pronation of the foot but they should be light and flexible for activity. Walking on toes and heels in movement sessions, without shoes, could assist with the development of an alternative walking style for children with Down syndrome and discourage them from continuing with a 'slap slap' style foot-strike pattern. Arm swing rhythms and posture activities using marching patterns and games can also improve walking.

Running

Running is an extension of walking in that it has an airborne phase. Because the magnitude of impact of the foot to the ground can exceed three times the child's body weight, attention to this pattern is essential to prevent injury especially to the child's lower limbs. This activity requires lower limb strength, balance, and good motor co-ordination for its mature form. For children with Down syndrome, movement experiences can make improvements in the support and flight phase, recovery phase and the arm actions. Speed should not be the primary objective.

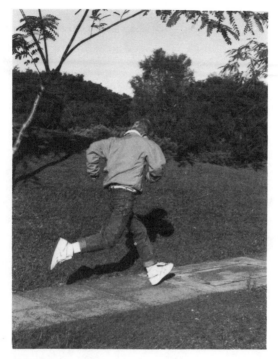

Figure 6.4 Energetic running.

Jumping

Jumping is an exciting skill to teach as there are so many variations of the basic skill. The child's first experience of jumping is descending stairs. Hopping is a form of jumping, in that it is a propelling force from one leg to landing on the same leg. If the child lands on a different leg, then it is a leap. We can jump forward, backward, up, down, around and sideways. Numerous additional pieces of equipment can be used to extend and vary practice opportunities. Games and sports are full of challenges for this skill.

DiRocco *et al.* (1987) studied the standing jump of children who were from four to seven years of age. They found that the group of children with mild mental retardation showed basically the same pattern of arm and leg co-ordination as the

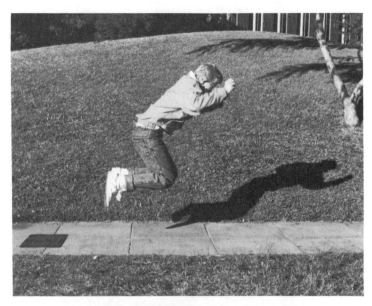

Figure 6.5 A jumping challenge.

comparison group, although arm actions were somewhat delayed. With regard to the performance aspect of the jump (i.e. the distance jumped), however, there was a lag of two or more years. This supported proposals (e.g. Davis, 1986) that the motor deficits in children with intellectual disabilities originate in control rather than co-ordination.

Throwing

Throwing is a most complex skill. It broadly has three basic phases: the preparation to ascertain the intended line of projection, the execution to determine the style (e.g. overarm) and direction of the throw, and the follow through and release of ball or object. With this motor skill pattern there are large sex differences (Haubenstricker *et al.*, 1983) but experience seems to play a significant role in improving the motor skill pattern in terms of distance, accuracy and speed. Children with Down syndrome require numerous and varied opportunities to practice this motor skill as it has relevance for their participation in many social games.

Catching

Catching involves the individual in bringing an airborne object under control using hands and arms. Early experiences for children with Down syndrome or those with slower development may involve trapping a ball rolled along the floor or table, or hugging a large ball. The mature performer predicts the flight and speed of a thrown object by adjusting the position of the arms and hands. 'The overall impression

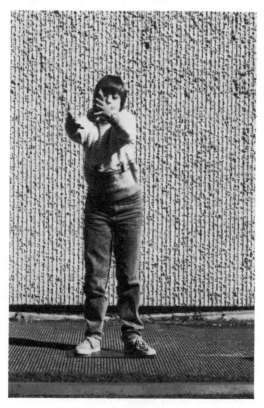

Figure 6.6 Preparing to catch the ball.

is of smoothness and ease. The eyes concentrated upon the ball; they do not watch the hands.' (Payne and Isaacs, 1991, p. 269).

Many movement experiences for children with Down syndrome can be devised using small equipment such as bean bags in playgrounds and floating objects in swimming pools to develop and improve this motor skill pattern.

PROGRAMMING CONSIDERATIONS

What rewards are there in movement for children with Down syndrome and how are they maintained?

The beginning walker is likely to persist if the pain of the constant falling is not perceived as too unpleasant in comparison with the adventure and enjoyment of exploring the environment. As young children progress toward middle childhood, they are most likely to choose to be involved in those physical experiences which have been enjoyable and which have given them a sense of competence.

In response to the question 'Why participate?' a large sample of elementary school children questioned by Gould (1984) gave these six reasons in their order of importance:

1. to have fun;
2. to improve skills and learn new tasks;
3. to be with friends and make new friends;
4. for thrills and excitement;
5. to succeed and win;
6. to become physically fit.

If long term and positive participation in activity for children with Down syndrome is the aim, then it is critical that the movement experiences in any program are enjoyable and will enhance skills.

These two aspects identified by children themselves then contribute to the other benefits of physical activity:

1. fitness;
2. effective and efficient movement;
3. confidence and positive self concept;
4. weight control;

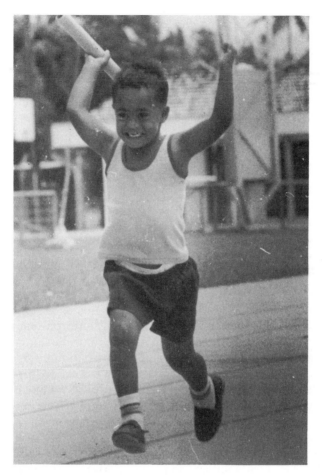

Figure 6.7 Success and excitement.

5. ability to utilize a variety of leisure options;
6. friendships – social context in teams, clubs and groups.

How then should programming help children with Down syndrome so that they *choose* to become physically active?

MOVEMENT EDUCATION

It is suggested that a movement education approach may provide the children with an avenue to express themselves, to learn, to explore, and challenge their own capabilities. The children are helped to understand movement from a mental, emotional and physical point of view (Laban, 1963; Morison, 1969; Laban, 1971; Fowler, 1981).

'It simply cannot be stressed strongly enough that even retarded children should be given an explanation for why they should do this or that . . . for if not the child will see no reason for his actions and will lose interest' (Holle, 1976, p. 144). The focus is on the feelings, ideas, abilities and interests of the children and the sessions are developed at the child's pace.

Children's own experiences can include:

Watch how I move and do this with me.
See the effect my moving can have on the world and others.
Look as I stand tall, or as I roll up tight and small.
Here is my foot, see how it stamps.

These experiences and others develop understanding of 'Do you move as I do?' and movement remains as an enjoyable activity to develop competence for long term participation.

To put oneself at the children's level, to understand them, their moving, and their needs requires much thought but these are essential components of a movement education approach. The teacher or therapist using this approach helps children to develop an awareness of the body in movement, a feeling for the movement in a kinaesthetic sense, and promotes the acquisition, development, and understanding of physical skills. Thus children are helped to gain insights into their own interests and capabilities. As Langendorfer (1985) suggested, such an approach to learning and teaching, with a focus on development shifts the emphasis away from the inabilities of the mover to an emphasis on the mover's uniqueness, competencies and abilities.

In a movement education approach, the physical activity programmes for young children with Down syndrome, can retain playfulness of movement, spontaneity, challenge, and initiative. Children can be given the opportunity to experience control and individual mastery. With a variety of exciting environments, materials and equipment, movement education can incorporate the 'resort model' approach for the therapist (Lyons, 1986; 1987) as well as involving physical education activities such as those suggested by Howe (1988), Sherborne (1990) and Stewart (1990).

The equipment and toys do not need to be expensive or sophisticated but variety can stimulate children to be interested in movement. Activities with equipment such as a colourful parachute have often been chosen (Carleton, 1989). The programme can also use everyday objects such as scarves, bean bags, hoops, bands, boxes, tin lids, water and sand. Children with Down syndrome may need to spend longer at a particular stage or task and could become bored with the same toy or piece of equipment. Toy libraries, if available, can help to extend the variety of equipment available.

A movement education approach makes allowances for the wide range of individual differences in the children's motor abilities. A balance can be maintained that facilitates enjoyment between the individual's skill level and the challenge of the activity, i.e. 'flow' in Csikszentmihalyi's terms.

Holle (1976) has suggested that 'the wish to participate should not be spoilt by making the task too difficult; ... experiences of progress and success will motivate children to continue.' (p. 163).

Children with Down syndrome may not learn movement tasks as readily as other chlidren. The teacher or therapist should therefore assist them to solve movement problems in the context of the movements that they can perform (Sherborne, 1982; 1990). Care must be taken that the movements are safe for those few children with atlanto-axial instability. Within the tasks, the movement qualities may demonstrate variability, lack of adaptation, and an inadequate knowledge of the movement requirements. A movement education approach to programming would provide the children with task variation, and a variety of opportunities to learn and to practise. It is not a training programme of constant repetition, so producing boredom and frustration, but it is an enjoyable and challenging style of teaching that assists understanding and knowing about the body and how it moves. As Sherrill (1988) has suggested, if practice is the prime ingredient for children with intellectual disabilities to improve their motor skill abilities, then the way we deliver that practice is critical.

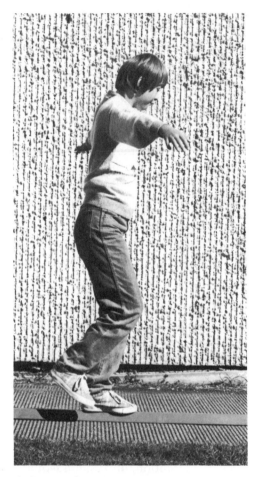

Figure 6.8 A balance task.

Another feature of this approach is its emphasis on the teacher's observation of the child's current movement qualities, abilities and experiences. The child's body and its movements are regarded as a communication system. On recognizing this communication, the teacher and peers can modify and extend the demands of the task and the situation to suit the child as an individual or as a member of a group.

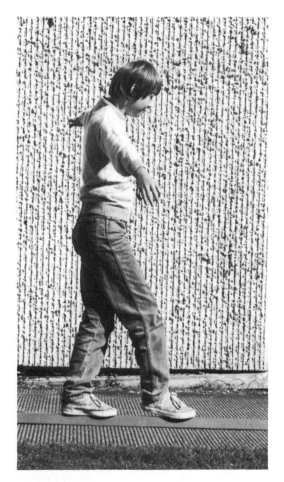

Figure 6.9 A balance task.

MOVEMENT SESSIONS

'At the preschool level movement work needs to co-ordinate and be concurrent with other teaching.' (Holle, 1976, p. 142).

Movement sessions whether co-ordinated with other aspects of the child's programme or not, need not be mindless repetitions of the movements to be learnt. They should be fun, allowing and providing a variety of experiences, so that the children can learn to move and to think about their movements.

Movement is a language of expression and communication and children need to understand:

1. what is moving? – body awareness;
2. where is it moving? – space awareness;
3. how is a movement made? – its flow, weight and time.

Movement experiences that include these Laban concepts give children an expanded repertoire of movement which they can interpret within a movement task or skill. Laban's language of movement provides the teacher with a wide variety of themes for movement. These themes concentrate on the childs's specific movement requirements for a task rather than on the skills needed to play a particular game. The children are encouraged to develop a quality in their movements as they associate space, weight, time and flow to parts of their body while moving. The themes can assist children to become more proficient in moving as well as providing a diversity of movement opportunities.

A session format

Sessions need to centre around the development of a movement theme. These themes are not imposed but developed within a framework of the children's movement abilities and interests. They should be designed to give the child variety, confidence and competence in moving.

Any session needs to commence with general movement and warm-up, followed by specific movement preparation or focus leading to a game, activity or dance. The general movement plan in a session should be designed so that energetic and less energetic movement activities are alternated and different muscle groups are used in rotation to prevent the children tiring and losing interest. Relaxation and stillness should be included in every session as the release of tension in muscles and an awareness of their breathing are valuable movement experiences for the children. Where tasks have to be repeated frequently or practised often, lessons can vary the speed, direction, sequence, body parts and equipment used to prevent boredom. They may also be taken in a different

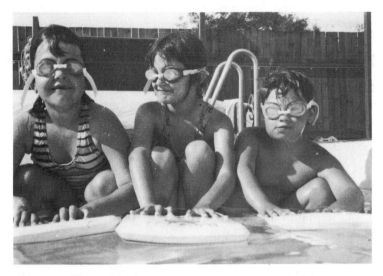

Figure 6.10 The swimming session.

environment e.g. moved from the playground to the pool or from the pool to the gymnasium.

The clothing and footwear worn by the children in the movement session needs careful consideration. Children cannot move freely and safely when encumbered with too much clothing and unsuitable, ill-fitting footwear. Everyday clothing may restrict mobility and become entangled in equipment causing injury.

Movement with language and drama

There may be a story book or a character from a book that is popular with the children, and movement ideas can be developed from these and used by the teacher. For instance, Winnie-the-Pooh characters – Tigger is a *bouncing* friend while Eeyore is *slow* and grumpy.

There are words that are associated with locomotion, gesture, and stillness. These can be used to explore movement sequences either within a category, such as locomotion e.g. 'run', 'hop' and 'jump', or in a combination of categories, such as locomotion, gesture, and stillness e.g. 'leap', 'reach' and 'freeze'. These word and movement 'games' are unlimited. Dramatic effects can be obtained by using percussion instruments or music.

It can be fun to use mime and gesture or other movements to practise sounds in action words, such as 's' in words like squirm, swish, slip, swing, slide and slither or 'f' in words like freeze, fly, flip, fling, flop.

Movement with mathematics

The content of this subject provides many opportunities to use movement as the motivator or stimulus for the learner to relate to mathematics and the body (Cratty, 1974; Dienes, 1973):

1. hopscotch and counting;
2. measurement and proportion;
3. shapes and size.

Movement with art, colour and shapes

Movement can provide a support in the teaching of colours and shapes and to discriminate differences. It can assist in the development of aesthetic awareness and the art's visual forms of line, colour, shape, texture and pattern.

Colours and shapes can be used to represent certain movements:

1. red as fiery, fast and flashy;
2. blue as cool, quiet and soothing;
3. squares as solid, and stable;
4. circles as moving and interacting.

Colours can be used to represent a team or group or to indicate the start or finish of an activity. In dance and marching activities, it is often helpful for the children to use colours to assist them with the directions and patterns of the required movements.

Movement with music

The combination of movement and music can assist children to explore, understand and interpret for themselves the 'space', 'effort', 'time' and 'flow' in their moving. It develops concepts such as sequence, rhythm and dance. These experiences may assist timing in other motor skill tasks and add variety and excitement to moving.

1. **Dance** can be folk, creative, exploratory, and with equipment, for example, ball, rope or hoop.
2. **Singing games** – 'You put your right hand in'; 'Johnny works with one hammer'.
3. **Free expression and creativity** – Carnival of the Animals, Pink Panther, Peter and the Wolf, Scott Joplin for creative expression.

Movement outdoors

Orienteering, simple map reading and compass skills are enjoyable activities that can be associated with movement experiences such as walking and climbing. They also provide a basis for later learning of skills necessary for the independent use of community facilities and negotiation of transport/travel. Activities which provide experiences in scrambling, rolling and sliding on grassy or snowy slopes, rough and tumble play on land or in the water and the digging, moulding and piling of sand or mud can be great fun. Chasing and dodging games outdoors can be not only fun but give children the opportunity to practise and improve locomotor skills. Camping, canoeing, sailing, fishing, and bush walking provide many movement education opportunities and the thrills of an adventure.

Movement with human relationships

Activities in which children learn about how their body works and about their relationship to others include body puzzle games, and relationship play. For example, in relationship play, a pair of children can face each other while holding hands and moving in a see-saw action (Sherborne, 1990). Working with a partner can be developed towards working in threes, fours and eventually in class groupings. The co-operative aspects of partner activities and the development of rules in games can assist children to develop an understanding of teamwork.

Colourbands, ribbons and small bells or rattles are useful in helping children identify body parts and to create interest in moving. They can also be used to assist the children to distinguish right and left sides of the body. Supporting surfaces such as floors, walls and other people can heighten awareness of body parts with tumbling, rolling and curling activities. This is especially true for the central aspects of the body such as the trunk or the shoulders, as without an awareness of these the child's movements are somewhat disconnected.

The possibilities for the use of movement within the school environment are endless. Many activities can be jointly created by the teacher, therapist, parent and the children. They can be developed into a thematic context. The children may help to develop a circus, Disneyland, spaceport, or motorcross obstacle course in the classroom, gymnasium, playground or swimming pool thus creating a new and exciting movement environment.

The movement education approach to programming:

1. involves the child in the activity;
2. can make learning fun;
3. can add variety to the slower rate of skill acquisition;
4. can expand horizons and increase understanding;
5. can create new associations for the child.

If there is careful progression towards competence, which is enjoyable for its own sake, then confidence is likely to follow.

The role of parent, teacher, or therapist in the movement programme includes that of participant, facilitator and observer. These roles are essential in a programme of movement experiences for children whose movement abilities may be different and whose problems may be difficult to understand. The adult's observation and supervision of the group serves to help, guide and encourage the movement experiences. The teacher or therapist need not demonstrate all the movement components themselves. The children, assisted by the teacher and using a variety of individual, partner, small group and large group formations can be used for this.

The teacher or therapist must be continually aware of the quality of the movements that the children are developing. This is important not only in expressive dance or gymnastics but in games and activities such as swimming and climbing.

It is simply not good enough to accept low standards of proficiency (Williamson, 1988). To accept that the child can swim no matter in what manner is not helpful as inappropriate movements can hamper future development. The highest quality and efficiency in the basic movement techniques should be developed.

CONCLUSION

In the play of children with Down syndrome, movement and physical activity have not been considered previously to the same extent as other aspects of development, such as cognition and language. Movement for these children, however, provides them with the chance to learn new skills and to enjoy new activities. With a movement approach, the children are provided with opportunities to communicate, solve problems, and explore movement in an enjoyable atmosphere. These experiences may not only assist movement proficiency, physical fitness, and social skills but they may also enhance self confidence and self esteem. It seems that the enjoyment of movement experiences should be nurtured and the child with Down syndrome should be encouraged and challenged to continue developing these experiences throughout life.

7

Fine motor skills in the classroom

Jenny Ziviani and John Elkins

INTRODUCTION

Although the wide ranging demands of the school require social, academic and practical skills for successful student life, educational attainment is primarily determined by the ability to demonstrate verbally and/or through inscription the comprehension and assimilation of knowledge. Difficulty in the execution of fine motor tasks such as handwriting and typing may act as disincentives to the mastery of the content of the curriculum.

Handwriting is one of a number of perceptual motor skills which children are routinely required to learn and master in their progression through school. The complex nature of handwriting makes it particularly susceptible to dysfunction. Conceived in its broadest sense, handwriting performance can be affected by the nature and quality of instruction to which an individual is exposed as well as by specific individual characteristics such as intellectual integrity, sensory perception, motor planning and execution. As Smyth and Wing (1984) expressed it 'handwriting is clearly a skill that can be described at various levels ranging from the initial organization of ideas to be communicated, the generation of grammatical structure, the selection of words to convey meaning, the determination of letter sequences, through the appropriate placement of individual pen strokes on the page.' (p. 298).

The use of the keyboard in the form of either a typewriter or computer is becoming a familiar educational activity.

Various computer-based teaching programmes have been developed for use in many areas of a school curriculum. The typing of assignments and the use of computer programs to develop number and language skills are becoming common-place in the classroom. While keyboard skills are a valuable educational and employment asset, they often serve to supplement rather than compensate for handwriting.

HANDWRITING

The process of writing has been conceived as first determining the message to be relayed, then translating this message into appropriate linguistic or expressive segments. Finally, individual segments are realized as a series of efferent commands (Rosenbaum, 1991). Underpinning the execution of written language is the establishment of a set of rules and motor programmes which facilitate the rate of response. For example, most circular movements are produced in an anti-clockwise direction and writing generally progresses from left to right across the page.

There is a plethora of factors which could be postulated as impacting on the acquisition of proficient handwriting by children with Down syndrome. These include the motor deficits related to timing and precision that were delineated by Henderson (1987) and the sensory, perceptual, motivational and physical characteristics of these children that may further impact on motor proficiency (Gunn, Chapter 1). In addition to what may be considered syndrome specific characteristics, there are individual differences regarding conceptual knowledge, exposure to instruction, social and familial support and experiences, and environmental constraints that influence handwriting. How children learn to form letters and place words on a page depends upon the assimilation of instructional material. What they write and how often depends on experience and opportunities.

The child's facility with language is also of prime importance as vocabulary and the ability to structure text and sequence words correctly are the foundations of written language (Meyers, 1990). Delays in acquiring handwriting skills may be expected in many children with Down syndrome as delays in language production and structure have been reported (Miller, 1987; 1988). On the other hand, spoken noun vocabularies are often in advance of syntax and very young children can amass a large corpus of sight words in their reading vocabulary (Buckley, 1987).

Although it is recognized that spoken language provides a basis for written language, a reciprocal effect has been suggested in that written expression can augment the spoken language of those with delayed speech. It is thought that the written language provides a way of increasing the understanding of grammatical markers. It is these markers which tie words together into sentences and are characterized by short duration, reduced stress and low volume (i.e. words such as do, is, will; or word endings such as -s, -ed) (Meyers, 1988).

As the focus of this chapter is the development of handwriting and keyboard skills, it will suffice to say that general language knowledge will impact on the written performance of children with Down syndrome. Specifically, it can be argued that reduced confidence with language will limit children's motivation to write. Further, poor understanding of structure may result in inappropriate spacing between words and letters during sentence construction.

While children with Down syndrome attain the same developmental milestones, albeit at a slower rate, as do their non-disabled peers (Dyer *et al.*, 1990), the performance of complex motor skills is often difficult for them. Learning to write requires the processing of visual, proprioceptive and to a lesser extent auditory information. Furthermore, effector mechanisms such as motor planning and execution are reliant both on central processes and neuromuscular integrity. With this backdrop, a number of avenues whereby the acquisition of handwriting might be hampered can be identified. As far as structural physical defects are concerned, as long as those involving vision and hearing impairment are recognized, they can be treated and in most cases, rectified.

As for the somatosensory system, specifically proprioception, it is more difficult to reach a conclusion. In part this is due to confusion with terminology since 'haptic', 'tactile', 'kinaesthetic' and 'proprioceptive' are often used interchangeably (Anwar, 1983). When considering handwriting, kinaesthetic is the term which is most consistently reported and refers to the location of joints during movement. Kinaesthesis is thought to play a very important part in the acquisition of writing. Specifically, kinaesthetic memory is thought to impact on writing proficiency (Laszlo and Bairstow, 1985). The role of superficial tactile sensation is less clear. It may be that fine adjustments of writing implements are in part reliant upon finger and pad sensation for control. If children with Down syndrome have tactile and kinaesthetic difficulties, these may underlie the establishment of motor memories for handwriting and impact upon pencil manipulation. Henderson (1987) has convincingly argued, however, that the existing evidence is inconclusive regarding these difficulties.

As one moves on to consider the execution of handwriting, two aspects need to be discussed, motor programmes and neuromuscular and skeletal characteristics. Turning first to motor programmes, these have variously been described as a centrally stored plan of action or sequence of movements (Schmidt, 1988). Certainly handwriting requires the rapid retrieval of letter and word plans especially if speed is the desired outcome. While children with Down syndrome demonstrate that they can assemble the requisite movement components in the performance of many manual tasks, they do not appear to execute these within spatial constraints (Hogg and Moss, 1983). Therefore when considering writing, their pencil hold and movements may be comparable to non-disabled children but the suggestion is that spatial and other qualitative aspects of performance may differ.

Specific neuromuscular characteristics of children with Down syndrome may influence handwriting performance. Hypotonicity is well documented (Dubowitz, 1980; Morris *et al.*, 1982) and while its direct impact on handwriting performance is difficult to isolate, poor trunk and grip stability can be postulated. Further, findings of diminished grip strength (Morris *et al.*, 1982) and joint hypermobility can both be considered to influence pencil grips. There has been little suggestion that the actual hand size and skeletal structure of the hands of children with Down syndrome have any specific influence on performance. They may however, influence some qualitative aspect of grip.

Apart from a report by Seagoe (1964) and the diary of Nigel Hunt (1966), there are few records of the writing achievements of children and adults with Down syndrome. Even so, Nigel Hunt's father wrote in the preface to the diary that his son found typing much easier than handwriting. Also, except for Pieterse and Treloar (1981), there is little documentation of the acquisition of drawing and pre-writing skills such as copying shapes, tracing lines and words.

In order to provide some qualitative and clinical impressions of a little documented skill, a description of the handwriting of a sample of children with Down syndrome was undertaken.

Twenty-four children with Down syndrome, who were taking part in a longitudinal study of the development of children with Down syndrome, were interviewed and their handwriting and graphic skills observed. The children comprised 12 boys (mean age 10.75 years, standard deviation 3.39) and 12 girls (mean age 11.65 years, standard deviation 2.48). Seven children attended regular schools, 13 attended special schools and four attended both, usually being enrolled at a special school with a couple of days each week at a regular school.

Children were seen individually. The tasks which the children were required to complete consisted of the Handwriting Performance Test (Ziviani and Elkins, 1984) for which normative data was available on the basis of handwriting formation, size, alignment, spacing and speed. This was used as a means of providing a broad statement about the level of performance of the children. In addition to this a number of clinical observations were recorded which aimed to provide more qualitative information on the strategies adopted and processes involved when children were writing. In summary, these observations included postural aspects of head, shoulder and arm positioning; pencil hold and manipulation; upper limb muscle tone and grip strength. Additional information was sought from individual children regarding their perception of their own writing and their exposure to and facility with keyboard activities. This was supplemented by comments from parents and teachers. Where children had access to keyboard communication their abilities were observed while typing a passage on a word processor.

LEGIBILITY AND SPEED

Given the paucity of documentation of the writing of children with Down syndrome, the first undertaking is to report the

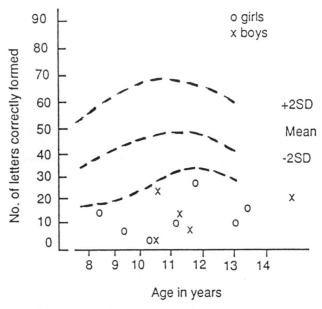

Figure 7.1 Letter formation.

performance of the children in this sample in relation to normative data for letter formation, horizontal alignment, consistency
of spacing, size and speed. As there were only 24 children in
this observation, these findings are reported diagramatically
rather than as statistical comparisons with the norm. Figure 7.1
summarizes the findings for letter formation. On the basis of
previous reports, it would be expected that children with Down
syndrome would have experienced greater difficulty than non-
disabled children. This was in fact the case for all the legibility
characteristics except for writing size, which, apart from three
girls whose writing was unusually large, fell within two standard deviations of the normative mean. Letter formation, the
characteristic which most strongly influences legibility (Mojet,
1991), fell below two standard deviations from the normative
mean for both girls and boys. This was also the case for the consistency of spacing between words. While it is not possible to
draw any statistical conclusions it would appear that the girls
in this group may have had greater difficulty maintaining
horizontal alignment of their writing than the boys.

The average speed with which children wrote was 29 letters per minute. This speed is less than that of an eight year old child without disability (Ziviani, 1984). Reports of reduced speed of performance are common in the literature on children with Down syndrome and therefore this finding is not surprising. Two observations were, however, inconsistent with the research on handwriting in children without disability. First, the correlation with age, while positive, was low (r = 0.40). Second, while in the general population girls have been found to write faster than boys (Ziviani, 1984), there was no significant difference between the boys and girls on writing speed (t = 0.17, df = 16, p = 0.86) despite a small but non-significant age difference of 0.9 years, favouring the girls.

PERFORMANCE CHARACTERISTICS

When interviewed all the children commented that they enjoyed writing and 21 (88%) stated that they were 'good writers'. These statements were not consistent with those of the children's parents or teachers who considered most of the

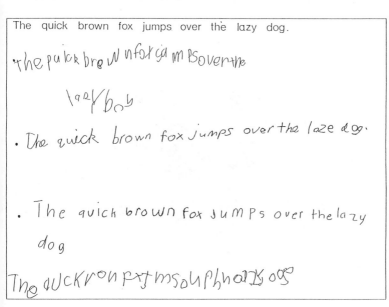

Figure 7.2 Variability in handwriting performance.

children to have writing difficulties. There is some evidence that children develop a concept of ability during the latter years of elementary school and the children in this study may be slower than usual in developing this concept (Stipek and MacIver, 1989).

Representative samples of writing (Figure 7.2) indicate the variability in performance which was encountered. In all, six children were unable to attempt the writing tasks. They were neither able to recognize the written symbols nor reproduce them.

Another five children were able to copy the required sentence but were unable to read it, leaving a little over half the sample of children able to both read and reproduce the sentence 'The quick brown fox jumps over the lazy dog.' In part, this is explained by the wide range of ages of the children. It also reflects, however, both a lack of familiarity with written symbols and uncertainty in their reproduction.

The way in which children wrote, while demonstrating individual variation, also showed some commonality. First with few exceptions children rushed to commence the tasks and after a short period of time demonstrated wandering attention which

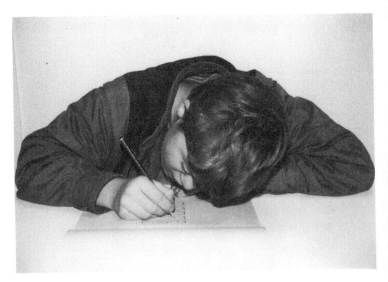

Figure 7.3 Sitting posture while handwriting.

was frequently accompanied by a slouching of their sitting posture. Postural control throughout was poor with children resting on their arms for support and dropping their heads (Figure 7.3).

This is consistent with the finding that all the children were clinically assessed as having slight to moderate hypotonia. In addition it was observed that a number of the children, as fatiguing became obvious, 'hitched' the shoulder of their writing arm. This was almost like a mechanical lock which could provide additional proximal stability.

Pencil grips adopted for writing exhibited a range of maturational levels and individual adaptations. A small number (three) used a dynamic tripod grip when writing. This involves the positioning of the pencil between the pads of the thumb and index finger while supported by the middle finger and allows the intrinsic muscles of the hand to control the fine movements of the fingers. This is the most developmentally mature grip which can be used for writing (Schneck and Henderson, 1990). The remaining grips employed can be divided into those which could be called less mature holds and those which represented an unusual adaptation of the tripod grip. Of the grips which can be called less mature, six children, primarily those below nine years of age, used a fisted grip

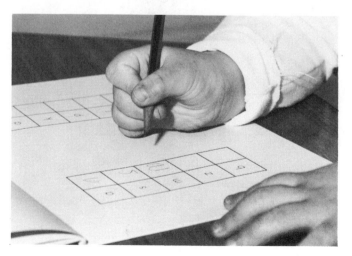

Figure 7.4 A fisted grip.

which involved the pencil being held in the thumb web space with the thumb and fingers curled around the shaft (Figure 7.4).

By its very nature this hold prevents intrinsic muscle action and relies upon wrist movements to complete a writing task. A further five children used a static tripod hold for writing. While the pencil is positioned as for the dynamic tripod grip there is little evidence of intrinsic muscle action and movement once again is primarily at the wrist.

The remainder of the children (n = 14) used adaptations of the dynamic tripod grip when writing. This is not an unusual occurrence as reports in the non-disabled population indicate that such variations may be quite functional (Bergmann, 1990). Variations in the non-disabled population have primarily been reported to consist of an increased number of fingers on the pencil shaft, lack of thumb opposition such as a lateral tripod hold, and hyperextension of the index finger. Most of the children with Down syndrome in the present group used thumb, index and middle fingers on the shaft of their pencils (Figure 7.5).

A few (n = 3) wrote with little stabilizing support from the little finger side of the hand resting on the page.

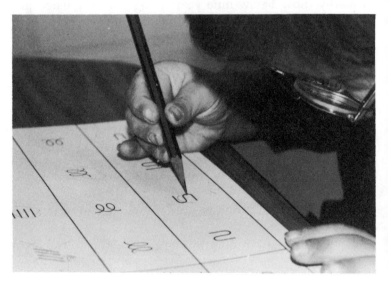

Figure 7.5 Thumb, index and middle fingers on pencil.

KEYBOARD SKILLS

Most of the children seen had received some exposure to the operation of a keyboard, fewer than half (n = 10), however, had the ability to reproduce text. For those who demonstrated this skill three were only able to do so through symbol matching leaving seven who could use the keyboard as an active means of communication. Four children who were able to use the keyboard for communication did so by finger typing. Many of the children used their middle fingers for typing, not favouring the index finger, as one would normally expect.

Often, the remaining fingers were held straight and not curled under as is normally the case with index finger typing. Typing was slow (11 letters per minute was the fastest that any of the children could type). Children spent considerable time scanning the keyboard to locate the right letters. Memory for letter positions seemed poor.

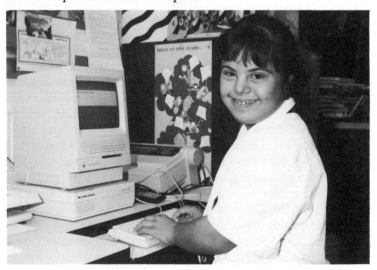

Figure 7.6 At the keyboard.

SUPPORT STRATEGIES

Handwriting and typing provide the chief methods of demonstrating educational attainments, as well as being assets socially and vocationally. It is obvious that these skills are complex and that some children may not acquire them. For those, however, who do demonstrate ability it is important that support be provided to facilitate successive stages of development.

There are a number of steps that need to be taken in investigating the difficulties encountered in the progression towards proficient handwriting or typing by children with Down syndrome. First the teacher must ascertain the existing stage of the skill and possibly seek further assistance from an occupational therapist or other professional who has knowledge about the development of skill independence. This type of consultation should allow the establishment of an individually tailored programme to help the child attain maximum proficiency.

This programme will be based on an assessment that considers four factors for each individual child. These include the child's knowledge of language (letters, words and sentence construction), the child's perceptual motor capabilities, the nature of any previous exposure to instruction and practice, and finally the child's motivation and interest in writing.

There is some research evidence which suggests that difficulty with language tasks may be evidenced in written form. Collette (1979) when examining children with dyslexia and reading delays found that they showed considerable variabilty in their letter size, reversals, and errors in forming loop letters. A profile, therefore, of reading and spelling as well as handwriting/typing ability is needed to ascertain whether a global or specific language skill is at risk for children with Down syndrome.

Assessment of perceptual motor competencies forms the second strategy when developing intervention programmes. Visual and auditory acuity as well as perception should be examined. In addition tactile and kinaesthetic sensitivity need to be considered, given the role of these systems in the acquisition of skilled movements (Laszlo, 1990). It is, however, kinaesthesis in conjunction with motor planning which seems to be most influential when considering handwriting (Copley and Ziviani, 1990; Laszlo and Broderick, 1991; van Galen, Meulenbrock and Hylkema, 1986). Activities that focus on copying continuous patterns of letters (either individually or joined into words) while directing the child's attention to what their movements feel like may assist in the refinement of kinaesthetic memory. Variation of demands to include change of size of writing may enhance motor planning of the task.

Postural low tone is evident when watching children with Down syndrome writing. Activities which involve joint compression (i.e. weight bearing such as wheelbarrow walking) or joint compression in addition to vestibular stimulation (i.e. trampoline exercises) are considered to be facilitatory to tone increase (Umphred, 1990). Undertaking these activities prior to tasks which require stable seating posture may be of assistance to some children. In addition manual activities which involve both compression and fine manipulation may also increase tone and joint awareness. Examples of these activities include construction tasks involving screws, nuts and bolts, pressing the parts together and paper tearing in collage projects.

The amount and nature of instruction received by children are known to influence the quality of handwriting performance (Sovik and Arnsten, 1991). Combining visual, verbal and kinaesthetic information when instructing in letter and word formation has been shown to be beneficial for children with intellectual disability (Vacc and Vacc, 1979).

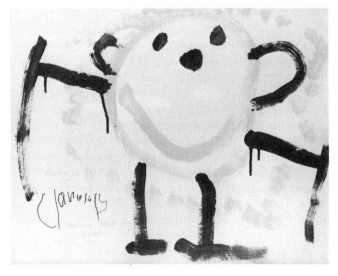

Figure 7.7 'Teacher' by Claire.

It is useful to remember that drawing is a developmental precursor to writing. Goodnow (1977) and Clay (1975) offer considerable insights into how children's drawing skills develop and how the representation of meaning through drawing leads to the use of graphic symbols for encoding language. The importance of encouraging students with Down syndrome to engage in drawing cannot be over-emphasized. Not only will they learn to control fine motor behaviour but they will also be led toward writing through such challenges as writing their name on the drawing and giving it a title (Figure 7.7).

Should students exhibit reverse letter ordering in such activities, it usually results from having begun to write too close to the right hand edge of the paper.

That school and home efforts are likely to produce benefits can be seen in the related area of musical and movement skills. Stratford and Ching (1989) noted that 'specific teaching approaches can significantly effect (sic) the development of children with Down syndrome in . . . music, movement and dance.' (p. 13). In the absence of detailed studies of instruction and encouragement in drawing and writing, it seems safe to recommend that attention be given to these areas by schools and by parents at home. To avoid age-inappropriate associations for older children, it may be important for teachers and parents to stimulate both drawing and writing topics which avoid 'childish' associations.

Irwin's (1989) study of school achievement indicates the benefits that can ensue not only from parents helping their child but also from encouraging schools to offer better curriculum opportunities. Thus we need to encourage schools which enrol children with Down syndrome to offer interesting and carefully structured opportunities to learn to write and type. There are a number of systematic teaching procedures for handwriting which might be tried with children who have Down syndrome. Most Australian states have adopted a linked script and have produced in-service packages to help teachers develop their skills in teaching handwriting. Similar developments have occurred in the United Kingdom (Carter, 1991).

Finally, individual motivation must be considered in every aspect of facilitating learning in children with Down syndrome, as with all children. Matching material to the child's capabilities is important when presenting any programme which then aims to extend these abilities. The use of micro-computers has been shown to be a useful adjunct to teaching children with developmental disabilities (Saunders, 1984) and can supplement writing and typing. Activities which involve symbol recognition and matching where children need to carefully examine and match shapes is a useful pre-writing exercise which may transfer to both manual and keyboard skills.

CONCLUSION

Drawing, handwriting and keyboard skills have not been given much attention by researchers interested in children with Down syndrome. Clearly more research on the development of drawing, handwriting and keyboard skills in these children is needed. Such an effort will be enhanced by close attention to the mainstream literature on these topics.

These are skills of great importance in their own right and because they enable cognitive activities to be carried out more efficiently. While the data presented in this chapter are limited, they illustrate that many children with Down syndrome can be taught these skills. There is, as in other academic areas, a good deal of variability among the students, with most having letter formation, size or fluency well below age standards. Despite this, their handwriting skills have functional value. They can draw pictures to illustrate their experiences and feelings, they can write stories and poems and can participate more widely in school curricula because of the tool value of these skills.

While the attainment of fluent, neat handwriting may be very difficult for persons with Down syndrome (as it is for many others), the computer and typewriter offer an easier path to the production of high quality graphic forms. The considerate teacher will recognize that it is possible to circumvent problems of slow or illegible handwriting by using word processing programs designed for novice writers, such as the Bank Street Writer/Speller.

While specific attention has not been given to Down syndrome, such students have been included in samples who have used computer-based writing instruction. Early studies were undertaken by Lally (1982) while Brewer and his colleagues have reported the use of a graphics tablet to shape fine motor control of handwriting (Brewer *et al.*, 1989/1990).

Parents and educators may need to advocate the provision of such aids so that students with Down syndrome are not unduly hindered in developing compositional skills. The acquisition of these skills clearly has significance for later vocational and social life.

8

Development of skills through adolescence and early adult life

Pamela Barham

Adolescence can be a pivotal time for people with Down syndrome. Learning to act positively and appropriately with peers and use community facilities independently is especially important to bridging the gap between adolescence and adulthood.

Feuerstein *et al.*, 1988 (p. 154)

INTRODUCTION

It is essential that deficiencies in the movement patterns of children with Down syndrome receive attention beyond childhood into adolescence (Harris, 1984). The quality of fundamental movements such as sitting, standing, walking and running require continued monitoring and physical fitness should be encouraged so that adolescents are helped to attain optimal motor competence. The progressive development of movement skills has the potential for enriching life experiences whereas body movements that are distorted, and/or unnatural are not only socially limiting for the young person with Down syndrome, but may be a cause of pain or injury.

Such limitations can become barriers to integration within the community and thwart attempts by adolescents and young adults with Down syndrome to become active participants in employment, leisure and recreational settings. The relationship of fine motor skills to vocational preparation has been mentioned in the previous chapter with respect to handwriting and keyboard use. These skills are important for proficiency in other settings. They are required for efficient performance on vocational tasks such as assembly work or machine maintenance. They are basic to many self-care activities (dressing, grooming, eating and cooking) and are essential for leisure pursuits such as fishing (baiting the line), craft work and gardening (planting and pruning).

There seems to be no study of employment tasks and motor proficiency relating specifically to Down syndrome but a study by Kerr *et al.* (1973) examined vocational programmes for adolescents with 'mental retardation'. This author recognized the importance not only of manual dexterity but also of balance, muscular strength and endurance but found little consideration of these attributes in school vocational programmes. The authors highlighted inconsistencies in adolescent performance and recommended that motor training programmes should be an integral and consistent part of the vocational education programme.

Recent reports about vocational programmes for adolescents with special needs have focused on the supported work model in which specific task skills are coached in actual working conditions. Although general motor proficiency and endurance may underpin success on these tasks, this is not widely acknowledged. There have been some suggestions, however, that there are more jobs for boys with intellectual disabilities than girls because of the need for physical strength and stamina in unskilled or semi-skilled jobs (McKerracher, 1984).

Just as there is limited data about employment and the motor proficiency of adolescents and adults with Down syndrome, there is also little information about the relationship between their motor competencies and activity choices. It has been reported, however, that the main activities of people with intellectual disabilities are passive and solitary in nature and that community recreational and leisure facilities are not used (Cheseldine and Jeffree, 1981; McConkey *et al.*, 1981). One reason which has been advanced to explain this non-participation is that the person is lacking in the skills required for participation. These skills include both those involved in the specific recreational activity, for example, techniques for playing specific games, and those needed to access community resources. Another suggestion is that the person has no friends with whom to participate. These suggestions have been supported in a study by Putnam *et al.* (1988) of 71 people with Down syndrome, from 15 to 31 years of age. It was found that 29% of the group lacked the skill to participate in a leisure activity and that 31% of the group had no-one to accompany them.

McConkey *et al.* (1981) concluded that leisure skills need to be taught in the same systematic and structured way as other areas of the curriculum if adolescents and adults with intellectual disabilities are to access community resources. A study by Weinberg (1981) with normally developing adolescents, however, is also relevant. He found that these adolescents participated in sports to have fun (90%), to improve skills (80%), to make friends (38%), and to become fit (56%). There seems to be no reason why adolescents with Down syndrome would participate for different reasons. That being so, we must ensure that the systematic structure ignores neither the opportunity 'to have fun' nor the opportunity 'to make friends'.

MOVEMENT EDUCATION

It is possible to design movement education programmes for adolescents and adults so that they provide not only systematic structure but also fun and social participation. These programmes give opportunities for exploring and mastering different movements in a variety of situations with the aim of expanding the person's understanding of their own movements.

The ability to observe movements accurately and sensitively is of paramount importance to the person guiding such a programme. Various aspects of movement management can be observed and these can provide consistent terms of reference to help participants to gain a better understanding of their own movements. Movement management includes the following seven aspects.

1. The anatomical mechanisms of the body, e.g. flexion, extension and rotation. These are frequently described in bodily terms as bending, stretching and twisting.

2. The type of activity, e.g. balancing, running and stopping, leaping, turning in the air and on the ground.
3. The parts of the body involved, e.g. the body parts leading or initiating an action like the body rotating before the release of the discus, or the body parts supporting weight or preparing to receive it, as in jumping.
4. The order in which different parts of the body are engaged, e.g. the sequential movements required to execute a basketball shot or the whole body responding at the same time, as in swimming.
5. The way the body is moving in terms of:
    Time – fast to slow movement;
    Weight – strong to light movement, the body weight distribution during movements;
    Space – generous or economic in the use of space, the space available in order to move safely;
    Flow – the quality of the movement demanded for a particular effort, free flowing or restricted, e.g. the strength required to kick a goal over a distance or the smooth even rhythm required to paddle a canoe.
6. The way the body is moving in space (in any direction), e.g. reaching into a cupboard while sitting in a chair, or running down an athletics track, or walking backwards.
7. The need for a person to move individually or with others, the size and structure of the group and the relationships within it, e.g. flying a kite alone, or square dancing with others, or the performance within a dance which may have one couple moving at a time or all dancers moving around in a circle at the same time.

Any intervention or verbal feedback from a teacher or therapist about home, job, or recreation-related movement will benefit from systematic observation of these aspects of management. For example, observation of an athlete throwing the discus, would involve:

1. which part of the body is mainly involved in the movement and in which direction is the body moving?
2. how much energy (force) is required to perform the movement?

3. how much pace is required?
4. how much control of the body is demanded to produce a good throw?

Movement education also includes practice in making decisions which are an integral part of movement proficiency. Opportunities for exploration in a wide variety of activities can help to give practice in such decision making.

One example is provided by Silk (1989) who structured activities for two groups of people with intellectual disabilities who were aged from 13 to 55 years. The activities were structured for self expression and decision making and the participants learnt how to extend their movement capabilities by:

1. creating dances in a large group after having made a collective decision about the music to be used;
2. adding additional movements one by one, e.g. a jump, a turn;
3. imitating one another's movements, usually working in pairs;
4. flowing movements into one another.

According to Silk, 'Exercises of this sort tend to build very strong non-verbal bonds between participants, and work well for both highly articulate and non-verbal clients.' (p. 57) This effect of movement development on relationships was also of prime significance to Laban (1963, 1971) and Sherborne (1982, 1990).

Laban believed that the 'feel' of a movement and the 'safety' of its continuous performance were of particular value. He stressed this self awareness aspect of movement through considering the qualitative components of time, weight, space, flow, and the inner feelings or attitudes associated with these components.

Sherborne (1982) emphasized this aspect when describing the way she introduced a movement experience programme to young persons with intellectual disabilities. For example, by using supporting surfaces, floor mats or the bodies of helpers, the participants learnt to roll on the floor or over a helper's legs, shoulders or back. Through practice in a variety of situations, both control and transfer of weight were experienced and the person concerned became fluent with movements associated with falling. The outcome of these experiences enhanced body awarenes and lessened fear of falling.

In Sherborne's (1982) view, through such experiences, a programme can contribute to the personal development of even those with the most severe handicaps. She believed that the experiences can foster both the development of a positive self image, and the development of the ability to form relationships. The provision of opportunities for social interaction and the growth of self confidence is indeed an essential component of a movement education programme.

Creating learning environments for adolescents and adults through the movement experience approach demands that the teacher works with the group, encouraging interaction and inventiveness. Use of props, hula hoops, scarves, balls of various size and weights, and coloured materials, assists participants to focus attention on the task in hand. By stretching to grasp hold of a thrown scarf, or spinning around in a hula hoop they become more aware of the body parts used, the need for body control, and the various contrasts in weight.

When teaching the skills of a ballgame, the body and ball must work in unison, therefore any activity which involves control of both is advancing an awareness of the demands on the individual. A teacher can encourage participants to exchange the ball from one hand to the other as the ball moves around their body, e.g. waist, hips, knees, ankles. Different ways of involving movement can be created by throwing or rolling the ball. Activities will come from the group as the session develops, as the participants become aware of their freedom, and as confidence in their own movement grows.

Children can be exposed to playgrounds with apparatus which encourages free flow experiences of swinging, sliding, and hanging. If children with Down syndrome have been assisted to swing, slide and roll, then as young adults they are more likely to have the confidence to respond readily and to lead others through creative movement sessions. A natural flexibility is a good starting point and with guidance and practice they develop more control of their balance and can become more competent in athletic activities.

In this book, Jobling has described experiences which may be incorporated into a movement education programme for young children. Some of these may be further adapted for adolescents and adults, for instance, the art, music and outdoor activities. The same principles can also be followed in adapting procedures for teaching team sport skills. One example is the following netball programme which has been undertaken with adolescents and young adults with Down syndrome. It has been found that individuals with various levels of ability can participate, enjoy and be extended by these activities.

A NETBALL PROGRAMME

The following programme is described as a practical illustration of the movement education ideas operating in the context of a team sport.

Theme: run, stop, and balance.
Equipment: hoops, bean bags, scarves, balls, coloured carpet squares.

Warm up:
1. Hoops are scattered around the space available and a scarf or a bean bag is placed in the centre of each hoop. The players transfer objects from one hoop to another moving as fast as possible.
   Alternatives:
   The distance between some hoops can be reduced.
   The players can work in pairs.
   The players work with a leader.
2. Hoops are set out as shown in Figure 8.1. The first player at hoop A picks up the object and moves as fast as possible to hoop B. A drops the object in the hoop and moves behind other players. This is repeated several times for each player.
   Alternatives:
   A variety of movements can be introduced e.g. walking briskly, long strides, side stepping.
   The distance between hoops can be shortened.
   Different equipment can be used, e.g. a ball instead of a scarf of bean bag.
   Hoop placement can be varied so that players follow a different path, e.g. circle, semi-cricle, zig-zag.

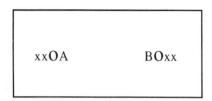

Figure 8.1 Warm up.

3. Each player sits in a hoop and draws one foot at a time into the hoop. The players raise the hoop above their heads using two hands. They turn sideways and back, then turn to the other side and back. This is repeated several times.

Skill development:
Hoops and players are positioned as shown in Figure 8.2.

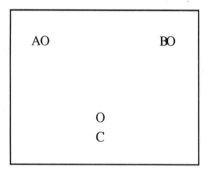

Figure 8.2 Skill development.

The player at A runs to B, catches the ball from the player at C. B then returns the ball to the player at C. Player C drops the ball in the hoop and then moves into the line behind A. The player at B moves to C. This can be repeated several times.
   Alternatives:
   Coloured carpet squares can be used instead of hoops.
   The distance between hoops can be varied.
   A roll or bounce pass can be used.
   Walking or slipping movements can replace running.
   The helper can replace the player at C.

A game situation

1. Five players and hoops are positioned on the court as shown in Figure 8.3 (players at positions A, B, C, D, E and hoops at A, B, C, D, E, F, G). The player C at the centre holds the ball.

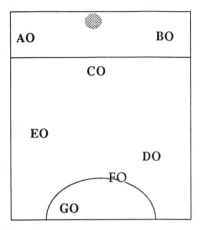

Figure 8.3 A game situation.

2. The first actions involve the players at A, B, and C. The player at C throws the ball to A (or B) and then moves to replace the player who did *not* receive the ball. This player moves on to the hoop at C in order to receive the next pass.
3. After receiving the pass, this player throws the ball to the player at D. At the same time, the player at E moves to G or F in the shooting circle.
4. The players then move form A, B, and C to E.
5. The player arriving first receives the pass. The other players move into the goal circle to defend.
6. The ball is thrown to player at G (or F) who attempts to score. Other players defend.

This routine is set up in groups of five at each end of a netball court and repeated several times.

Alternatives:
Coloured squares are used instead of hoops.
The positions for players to stand are varied, i.e. the player at the centre circle is the only moving players.
The centre player and others are interchanged.

Cool down activity:
Each person should stand in their own space on a mat or in a hoop on a court. The coach provides a model by clasping hands overhead and stretching up, forward and sideways.

Alternatives:
The positions are varied, i.e. to lying or sitting.

Combining basic skill movements in the 'run, stop and balance' activities can be helped by the use of portable

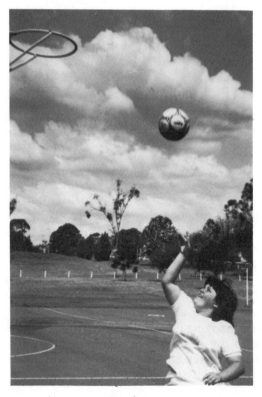

Figure 8.4 Netball success. (Reproduced with permission from Project Recreation, Ipswich, Queensland, Australia).

apparatus which is attractively presented. In the previous example, hoops, carpet squares, and markers were used as focal points for changes in an activity, e.g. from running to jumping and turning. They can be used also as focal points for changes in the direction of a movement, e.g. from travelling forwards to travelling backwards or sideways.

By adding a ball which has to be rolled around a hoop, bounced into a hoop, or thrown through a hoop, attention has to be directed towards stopping the ball. Techniques of catching or trapping, as in soccer need to be developed and the movements have to become more refined. The previous practices assist this development in interesting and structured ways and the writer has found them acceptable to many age groups.

Lead-up games to traditional netball can be easily introduced, with or without helpers, and young people with various levels of ablity can enjoy movement, competition and companionship with some degree of independence.

PHYSICAL FITNESS

In addition to the specific movement skills required for an activity, it is important to consider the physical fitness of the participants, both health-related and skill-related fitness. Following the description by Dyer and Berry (1991), health-related fitness is associated with attributes such as endurance, strength and flexibility whereas skill-related fitness includes attributes such as speed, agility, power, co-ordination and balance. An adolescent with a low physical fitness level will find it difficult to keep up with the pace of many recreational activities. Indeed, it can be argued that any skill-based programme, whether structured to improve work, sport or recreation activities, will be limited if attention is not given to the level of physical fitness. As Kelly *et al.* (1986) stated, ' . . . it is counter-productive to develop vocational and recreational skills of mentally retarded individuals while at the same time ignoring factors such as obesity and fitness that will ultimately limit the ability of these individuals to use their skills to their maximum potential.' (1986, p. 174).

There is general agreement that there is a relationship between obesity in Down syndrome and level of fitness although the reporting is often limited in terms of the size of the sample studied and the methods used for measurement and assessment (Kelly *et al.*, 1986; Seidl *et al.*, 1987, Pitetti *et al.*, 1988 and Pizarro, 1990). An early onset of obesity in children with Down syndrome has been reported clinically but is poorly documented (Cronk *et al.*, 1985). This is of concern as childhod obesity has been shown to lead to adult obesity (Burkart *et al.*, 1985). Johnson and Werner (1980) have graphically described the consequences of obesity for daily functioning, ' . . . he may be so obese that such simple routines as walking, bending over, carrying a lunch tray or getting into a car are extremely difficult.' (p. 129).

Weight gain is the outcome of an imbalance between caloric intake and energy expenditure, therefore attention to both diet and exercise is needed when addressing this problem. According to Emes *et al.* (1990), an inactive lifestyle is more characteristic of obese adolescents than overeating. Chad *et al.* (1990), however, came to the conclusion that an examination of the metabolic rate in relationship to diet, and anthropometric measures, were needed to assess the association between activity and weight gain for children with Down syndrome and Pueschel (1987) cautioned that obesity in either adolescence or adulthood may be related to hypothyroidism.

It has been suggested that activity programmes requiring gross motor and large muscle group movements that are presented regularly over several weeks will help to reduce obesity and improve the fitness of participants with Down syndrome (Mulholland and McNeill 1985; Dyer and Berry, 1991). There are several studies of activity programmes for adolescents and young adults with intellectual disabilities that are relevant to Down syndrome. Beasley (1982) found that a jogging programme improved both cardiovascular fitness and work performance while Ginn (1988) reported that a programme which included aerobic fitness, anaerobic fitness, flexibility and strength was beneficial to stamina and the standard of ball-game play.

Corbin and Lindsey (1984) have analysed a variety of sports and exercise programs for their health-related benefits, cardiovascular fitness, development of strength, muscular endurance and flexbility, and control of obesity. Among the activities that were rated highly were several which would be enjoyed by young people with Down syndrome. These included bicycling, swimming, cross country skiing, dancing, various football codes and basketball. Bicycling, swimming, and cross country skiing were rated as excellent for both fitness and control of obesity. Basketball and soccer were given an excellent rating for fitness and were rated as good for obesity control. It must be noted, however, that soccer and other high body contact sports are not suitable for those with atlanto-axial instability.

An additional benefit noted by Corbin and Lindsey is the suitability of some of these activities for lifetime pursuits. Several other activities which also have the possibility for lifetime interest were given fair or poor ratings regarding their health benefits but their potential for personal enjoyment or for socialization should not be forgotten. These activities include bowling, canoeing, skating and horseback riding although for those with atlanto-axial instability, horseback riding is not recommended.

It may be noted also that some activities require well developed perceptual or decision-making skills. For those learners who have difficulty in acquiring these skills, activities such as swimming, hiking, and creative dancing may be suitable alternatives. Fitness exercises are easily adapted to the capabilities of even the slowest learner and are an important component of activity programmes.

FITNESS EXERCISES

The presentation of these exercises is important and motivation by the facilitator should be expressed in both voice and action. It would be advisable for the initial activities to be simple with frequent demonstrations and verbal cues kept to a minimum. The language should not be complex and the directions should be concise and given in a motivating manner. For example, sharp, quick speech can be used to give 'jumping ... go!' directions but slow, drawn out speech would be used for 'slow...ly, str...etch' type directions.

Action is the key and the use of action-orientated words will help to keep the movements going at a steady pace. For example:

JOG along the lines of the area;
JUMP over the rope;

SLIP along this line;
SPRINT back to your place;
STOP and rest.

The recreational space should look inviting with bright coloured markers as turning points, especially if the activities are being undertaken in a large space. For example, hoops may be used to run over or around, witch's hats are suitable for jumping over or slipping around and cones can be used to indicate that a change in action is required.

The participants should be kept active over the number of repetitions required and they should be sweating lightly at the end of the warm-up activities.

Stretching exercises should be simple but varied and the teacher needs to be perceptive about the way the participants are performing these exercises.

It is advisable to demonstrate while drawing attention verbally to the parts of the body involved. Some examples include 'wrist flick', 'toes curl', 'arms swing', and 'bend slowly sideways – feel the stretch in your side.' Such a stretching exercise routine follows the Laban principles of movement education through its role in increasing each participant's body awareness of time, weight, space, and flow.

Each fitness component should be scheduled into the routines. Some elements can be developed together. For instance, mobility and aerobic fitness components can be presented by a running weaving pattern around markers, even though only one marker may be used for the less able participants. The fitness levels of the players can be improved by increasing the rate of exercise and the intensity. Ten seconds of hard exercise is sufficient, followed by 30 seconds of recovery type movements such as jogging around the space being used, or throwing a ball to a partner while moving slowly around a specified space. Explosive power and anaerobic work can be included in strength training programmes and these provide several levels of participation through height and weight differences.

The difficulty of the routines can be varied to suit the understanding of the participants and to match the various levels of experience. Several different activities can be undertaken simultaneously in the form of a circuit. The exercises

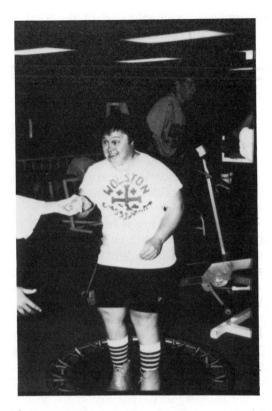

Figure 8.5 Becoming fit. (Reproduced with permission from Project Recreation, Ipswich, Queensland, Australia).

should be repeated for several sessions so that familiarity of the routine allows for improvement in the intensity of participation.

Fitness programmes should include fun activities, e.g. obstacle circuits and relay games. These games should alternate fast rowdy activities with the more concentrated, or slow, balancing types of activity. It will of course be necessary to take into account any heart or health problems of the participants.

The cool down period is an essential part of the activity session. It assists in the physical toning of the body and acts as a quiet activity for the participants. A period of relaxation and stillness is also a valuable part of the total movement experience.

PROGRESSIVE PROGRAMMING

The desirability of ensuring some continuity in movement experiences from childhood to adolescence to adulthood must not be forgotten. Sport or recreational competencies developed earlier may be lost if there is no opportunity for further practice. If the young person with Down syndrome is encouraged to develop the skill and confidence to participate in a recreational pursuit, it is vital to consider also the possibilities for continuous participation.

If progressive programming is to be planned, there are a number of factors which should be considered. The primary need is to develop and maintain positive attitudes in all participants and this requires long-term planning and commitment. A most important requirement is that the young people have easy access to programmes that are offered on a regular basis. It is important that a choice of options should be available so that a variety of interests and abilities can be satisfied. This choice may be across different activities or it may involve the different opportunities for achievement which can be provided within the one recreational activity. These can range from the mastery of movement skills, to skill in both the movements and strategies of a team game, to achievement in the organization of games or to recognition as a scorer or umpire.

Several other factors need to be considered when planning on a long-term basis. These include the possibility of obtaining professional assistance from community groups, the units of time and the budget available, the location of facilities and equipment (whether segregated or integrated within the community), and the regular monitoring and evaluation of the programme. Quality in long-term programming can be achieved only by thoughtful planning and monitoring.

CONCLUSION

There are many possible benefits for adolescents and adults with Down syndrome from participation in regular movement activities. These include weight reduction and control, an increase in motor proficiency, the development of confidence, a positive self concept and the ability to use leisure time in a positive and healthy way (Sim and Stewart, 1984).

The self-awareness benefits for those who take part in a movement education programme include an awareness of their own movements and capabilities and an insight into the changes that effort and practice can bring to movement skills. Further, their growth in self confidence may encourage them to choose an activity with the knowledge that they are competent to learn. They then have the opportunity of enjoying both the activity and the companionship of others who have the same interests.

Although the emphasis in this chapter has been on recreational aspects of movement education, it should be stressed that these programmes not only assist participation in recreational activities but also help to develop many of the motor competencies needed at home and for employment. Moreover, these experiences can be valued for their relaxation and enjoyment qualities as well as for their role in developing the physically fit and socially competent adult.

9

The elderly person with Down syndrome: the benefits of an active life

Barbara James

INTRODUCTION

Ageing is a complex phenomenon and is the result of a continuing interplay of both genetic and environmental factors, so that although there are common traits with respect to the age of onset of manifestations of the ageing processes, the rate of ageing varies considerably between individuals. To complicate the picture of ageing, one of the environmental factors which causes similar adaptations to 'ageing' per se is a decreasing level of physical activity. Levels of physical activity often decline with age but this may be caused in part by a lack of opportunity to participate in suitable leisure activities.

In many Western countries, there has been an increase in the opportunities for the general population to remain socially active, with a proliferation of clubs for 'senior citizens'. Clubs offering active recreation such as lawn bowls, croquet, exercise to music, and social dancing are readily available in many towns and cities. The stereotype of a person 'slowing down' on retirement (Bassey, 1978) is changing as people are now more aware of the necessity to remain active at all stages during life. These changes in attitude, expectation, and opportunities, allied with the expansion in the numbers of elderly persons with Down syndrome, make it timely to examine these trends in relation to the lives of adults with Down syndrome.

Appropriate and effective activity programmes for older adults can only be achieved with a cognizance of how the ageing processes affect functional capacity and how activity levels affect the functional characteristics. Characteristics of particular importance are motor performance and joint mobility, because changes in muscular strength, co-ordination and endurance, and the range of movement at the joints are central to the activities of daily living. Physical characteristics may be another important consideration in the population with Down syndrome because of the influence of body configuration on movement capacity.

Because ageing in the population with Down syndrome is not well documented, the following sections present information about the general population of older persons aged more than 65 to 70 years and where appropriate, about the population described as 'mentally retarded'. Although this age level is regarded as old in the general community, Down syndrome is characterized by an increased speed of ageing, including early menopause (Miniszek, 1983) and a better definition of 'old' for adults with Down syndrome may be over 50 years of age (Seltzer, 1985).

MOTOR PERFORMANCE

Although a number of the body's subsystems underlie efficient movement, the neuromuscular system is particularly important because it is responsible for both the motor patterns and the postural or balance adjustments needed to prevent falls. The literature will therefore be reviewed on aspects of the neuromuscular system relevant to common movement functions.

Ageing adaptations in the neuromuscular system

A striking feature of ageing is the reduction in the skeletal muscle volume (Allen *et al.*, 1960; Tzankoff and Norris, 1977; Borkan *et al.*, 1985) which is caused by both a loss of muscle fibres (Lexell *et al.*, 1983; Sato *et al.*, 1984, 1986) and by muscle fibre atrophy (Essen-Gustavsson and Borges, 1986; Brown, 1987). An important effect of ageing is that differential changes occur in the composition and volume of the different muscle fibre types. The physiological properties of the two basic fibre types, I and II, can be summarized as follows: type I are innervated by frequently active motoneurons that can fire at low frequencies and have slower conduction velocities. These muscle fibres show less fatigue, and can sustain tension for longer periods of time. Type II fibres are innervated by less active motoneurons that can fire at high frequencies and have fast conduction velocities, but maintain activity only for short periods. These muscle fibres develop tension rapidly and can maintain it only for short periods of time (Kovanen, 1989). There is a more pronounced loss of type II fibres than of type I fibres with increasing age (Lindboe and Torvik, 1982; Oetel, 1986; Sato *et al.*, 1986), and fibre diameter decreases to a greater extent in type II fibres (Scelsi *et al.*, 1980; Sato *et al.*, 1984). Another common morphological change is the grouping of type I fibres in large clusters, whereas the two fibre types are organized in a random arrangement in young muscle (Aniansson *et al.*, 1984a; Brown, 1987). This happens because some type II fibres are converted to type I fibres. Although there is a gradual reduction in the motor unit number, there is an increase in size with the remaining units predominantly of the slow-twitch type (Campbell *et al.*, 1973; Stahlberg and Fawcett, 1982). As will be discussed in the next section, these adaptations favour muscular endurance.

There is a dearth of information on ageing in the motor system in Down syndrome, or even the wider mentally retarded population. Apart from the fact that ageing adaptations manifest in a 'premature and severe fashion' in intellectually disabled persons, it has been suggested that neuromuscular ageing does not differ from that of the general population (Rudelli, 1985). The presence of hypotonia, which may be present in some adults with Down syndrome, also does not show specific differentiating morphological features in the ageing of the motor system (Rudelli, 1985).

Performance characteristics

It is well established that there is a decline in muscular strength as people age, due to the decrease in the number of muscle fibres and functioning motor units, together with muscle fibre atrophy. Isokinetic strength deteriorates faster than isometric strength, particularly when measured at faster velocities (Larsson *et al.*, 1979; Aniansson *et al.*, 1983; Danneskiold-Samsoe *et al.*, 1984; Cunningham *et al.*, 1987). It has been hypothesized that this is a consequence of the preferential atrophy of type II fibres, because of the importance of these fibres during higher contraction velocities (Aniansson *et al.*, 1983).

Muscular endurance also declines during ageing (Shock and Norris, 1970). If a correction is made for the decrease in maximum strength, differences between young and elderly adults disappear (Aniansson *et al.*, 1978; Larsson and Karlsson, 1978). This has been attributed to the relatively greater proportion of type I fibres in older people which increases the ability to sustain tension. The fibre type reorganization favouring type I fibres will take place earlier in active people. Kovanen (1989) has suggested that this occurs in order to facilitate the performance of sustained work at a lower energy cost.

Most basic movement requires the co-ordination of the activity of a number of muscle groups, and depends not only on the force that can be exerted by the individual muscle groups involved, but also on the effectiveness of their co-ordination. It has been shown that the isometric strength of individual muscles does not decline as early as strength measurements involving a number of muscles (Shock and Norris, 1970; Larsson *et al.*, 1979). Movement quality may also be affected adversely with increasing age because of the reduced efficiency of proprioceptive mechanisms, resulting in an impairment of information transfer to the central nervous system to aid in movement control (Woollacott, 1986). Joint position sense, as determined by measurement of the threshold at which motion is detected, and the ability to reproduce joint position deteriorate with age (Skinner *et al.*, 1984; Kaplan *et al.*, 1985) and the perception of vibration in the feet and ankles worsens (Lascells and Thomas, 1966; Kokmen *et al.*, 1977).

In summary, a number of age-related changes in the neuromuscular system which affect functional performance have been identified. These include the decline in muscle strength of muscle groups and the impairment to co-ordination. This is manifested in greater deficiencies in isokinetic than in isometric strength (Larsson *et al.*, 1979; Aniansson *et al.*,

1980, 1983; Murray *et al.*, 1980). The control of dynamic balance is also important in many activities, and deficiencies in such factors as joint motion sensation and perception may be important in this respect. Since the ankle joint in particular is a major source of receptors controlling posture, this loss would be expected to decrease balance control (Woollacott, 1986) and so have important implications in activities involving the upright posture.

There seem to be no reports concerning changes in motor performance with increasing age in Down syndrome. At younger ages this group generally shows reduced motor performance and there is no reason to believe that ageing changes would not parallel the morphological changes as in the general population. The process and consequences of motor system ageing among people with Down syndrome, however, is an area that warrants greater consideration and research.

JOINT MOBILITY

Another functional characteristic of particular interest in the activities of daily living is the range of movement at the joints. Joint mobility is not a stable characteristic during adulthood in the general population, and limitations may contribute to modifications in the movement patterns required in self-care activities such as reaching to high shelves or tying shoe laces, and gross motor activities like walking (Murray *et al.*, 1969) and stair climbing (James, 1991).

Ageing adaptations in joint function

Age-associated alterations in joint function occur basically because of modifications in joint structures (Huson, 1984). These are caused primarily by ageing changes in the morphology of joint tissues which act generally to reduce their compliance (Hall, 1976) and so cause greater resistance to deformation on movement. The geometry of the articulating surfaces also determines the degree of mobility of a joint (Huson, 1984), and the remodelling of articular surfaces throughout life results in an increasing congruity between the articulating joint surfaces particularly in weight bearing joints (Bullough, 1981). This results in increased active resistance where bony surfaces come into contact at the extremes of movement (Walker, 1977).

Remodelling of the articular surfaces also occurs as a result of degenerative joint disease such as osteoarthritis (Sokoloff, 1969; Allander *et al.*, 1974) and is thought to cause increased limitations to joint mobility. Trauma-related joint pathology may also contribute to variability in joint motion. Repetitive damage over the years results in modifications to cartilaginous and tendinous joint structures which restrict joint motion (Allander *et al.*, 1974). Similar effects may result from maladaptive movement patterns in people with Down syndrome over time.

Changes in joint mobility also occur in response to different functional states (Hall, 1976). Repetitive use of specific joint movements or activities (Leighton, 1957; Kuta *et al.*, 1970) and customary postures (Walker, 1975) cause alterations in structures which reflect the tensions to which they are habitually subjected. Physical activity is important for retaining the biomechanical characteristics associated with normal function in synovial joints (Akeson *et al.*, 1987), because loading of the articular surfaces is necessary in providing the stimulus for the nourishment of peri-articular tissues.

On the other hand, inactivity is suggested as a detrimental influence on the passive elongation properties of muscle (Halar *et al.*, 1978). Adaptations in the joint capsule occur with immobilization or the use of restricted ranges of movement (Johns and Wright, 1962; Williams and Goldspink, 1984; Savolainen *et al.*, 1988). Muscles habitually worked at a shortened length also showed a loss of sarcomeres and reduction in muscle fibre length (Williams and Goldspink, 1973), thereby contributing to reduced functional joint ranges.

A number of studies over wide age ranges indicate increasing limitations with age from the early adult years (Allander *et al.*, 1974; Boone and Azen, 1979; Bell and Hoshizaki, 1981; Boone *et al.*, 1981). Investigations of older adults also show an ongoing reduction in mobility from middle age (Smith and Walker, 1983; Walker *et al.*, 1984; James and Parker, 1989). There is some specificity in this reduction of joint movements. For example, upper limb joint mobility decreases more than lower limb joint mobility (Allander *et al.*, 1974; Bell and

Hoshizaki, 1981; James, 1983). Bell and Hoshizaki (1981) attribute this to higher levels of activity involving the upper limb throughout life. More importantly, it is likely to reflect structural adaptations in the lower limb joints in response to weight bearing.

Mobility in Down syndrome

Hypermobility is one of the common characteristics of Down syndrome children, however, little has been documented on changes in mobility during the adult years. Ankle dorsi-flexion with the knee in extension is the only motion studied in a wide age range, and no evidence was shown in these subjects aged 17 to 60 years of hypermobility (Mahan *et al.*, 1983). The primary cause of hypermobility in children with Down syndrome has been attributed to hypotonia but this condition seems to improve during the developmental years. There is some evidence of the specificity of joint mobility in the population with Down syndrome, with the hip being more affected than the other joints (Bennet *et al.*, 1982; James, 1983). Subjective observation suggests that this greater mobility in hip joint movements may persist during adulthood.

PHYSICAL CHARACTERISTICS OF OLDER ADULTS

Alterations in the size, shape and proportions of the body are readily observed during ageing, and this may have implications for some movement functions (Stoudt, 1981). Men and women decrease in height with increasing age (Damon *et al.*, 1972; Dequeker *et al.*, 1983) primarily because of skeletal changes in the anatomic length of the vertebral column resulting from thinning of the intervertebral discs (Twomey, 1981), and postural adaptations (Stoudt, 1981). Body weight generally increases in response to increased nutrition and/or decreased activity levels.

The major tissues of the body vary considerably with age resulting in changes in body composition (Chumlea and Baumgartner, 1989) and of the three tissue groups, fat shows the greatest change (Skerlj, 1959). The lean body mass declines with age, primarily through atrophy of the skeletal musculature (Norris *et al.*, 1963; Forbes, 1976; Borkan and Norris, 1977).

In contrast, there is a tendency to increased fat deposition with advancing age (Skerlj *et al.*, 1953; Krzywicki and Chinn, 1967; Borkan and Norris, 1977).

People with Down syndrome are characterized by their shortness of stature, which is due predominantly to a reduced length of the lower limbs (Rarick and Seefeldt, 1974), and by their higher percentage of body fat (Bronks and Parker, 1985). There appears to be no difference in the basal metabolic rate in healthy adults with Down syndrome (Schapiro and Rapoport, 1989), and it has been suggested therefore, that along with diet, a regime of daily physical activity which increases the metabolic rate during, and for a considerable period of time following exercise cessation should help in decreasing obesity (Chad *et al.*, 1990).

In summary, there are age changes in body mass distribution, with the upper body becoming a relatively larger proportion of the total. These changes indicate differences in the inertial characteristics of the body which suggest an increased instability with possible implications for dynamic postural control. In people with Down syndrome, however, movement capability may be compromised more by obesity than by changes in body mass distribution. This may be reflected in a greater physical effort to move the body, and in the effects on the lower limb joints during standing and locomotor activities.

FUNCTIONAL CAPACITY AND ACTIVITY

Alterations in the neuromuscular system with increasing age have a complex aetiology related both to intrinsic and environmental factors. The complexity is increased because distinguishing between changes resulting from ageing per se and those attributable to pathological processes is difficult. It is also well recognized that disuse causes similar effects during the course of ageing (Froklis *et al.*, 1976; Gutmann and Hanzlikova, 1976). For example, changes in fibre type distribution in aged muscles may reflect changes in function. Activity patterns of older adults are much more limited than in the young, thus changing or decreasing the functional demands on the fibre type population, with respect to force, velocity, and duration. Endurance training was found to help maintain muscular performance by the promotion of changes in muscle fibres to increase resistance to fatigue and by improved mechanical properties in muscle (Kovanen, 1989).

Another way of examining the relationship between activity and neuromuscular system function is to compare groups with different habitual activity levels, and a number of studies show that muscular strength is higher in those who regularly engage in physical activity compared to those who do not (Kuta *et al.*, 1970; Kroll and Clarkson, 1978; Aniansson *et al.*, 1980, 1983, 1984b).

The benefits of activity on joint mobility also have been demonstrated. Older men (60 to 80 years) who had been active in sport or athletics during the previous decade showed increased joint mobility when compared with their sedentary counterparts (Kuta *et al.*, 1970). A survey of older women also indicated that those who attended yoga classes had retained excellent spinal mobility, while the less active women showed considerable losses (Rankine-Wilson, 1980).

At the functional level, it has also been shown that sedentary older people experienced an increased need of assistance in the activities of daily living, and greater difficulty in walking or climbing stairs than their peers who had previously been engaged in active manual work, or were at least moderately active in leisure activities throughout their adult lives (Bergstrom, 1985). The importance of physical activity was emphasized also in the positive relationship between habitual activity level and walking speed and stepping height capability in older men and women (Aniansson and Gustafsson, 1981).

With regard to adults with Down syndrome, it has been suggested that activity levels are likely to be reduced during old age, because of the passive nature of their everyday lives, and their dependence on others to meet daily needs (Ropper and Williams, 1980). Although no studies have been reported that compare the performance of daily living activities in older people with Down syndrome who have different habitual activity levels, it would be expected that findings in the general population could be extrapolated to these people. Also, it is expected that changes towards increased independence and a greater involvement in community activities would impact on the activity levels and functional competence of future generations of elderly adults with Down syndrome.

Response to training

A number of studies clearly show that the physical fitness of older people can be improved even though they may have been sedentary for many years. An increased economy of effort has been shown in older people after physical training (Skinner *et al.*, 1984; Tzankoff *et al.*, 1972; Suominen *et al.*, 1977; Sidney and Shephard, 1978; Aniansson and Gustafsson, 1981; Aniansson *et al.*, 1984a). Subjects were physically active for longer (Adams and de Vries, 1973), worked more vigorously (Skinner *et al.*, 1964), and both static and dynamic muscle strength increased with training (Moritani and de Vries, 1980; Aniansson and Gustafsson, 1981; Aniansson, 1984). Adaptive changes occurred in the muscle fibres, resulting in improvement in the co-ordination of the movement (Moritani and de Vries, 1980).

Advanced age in itself does not inhibit the capability of muscles and joint tissues to respond to changes in joint use. The effects of a training programme in producing changes in joint stiffness in men aged 63 to 88 years was compared with young men (Chapman *et al.*, 1972), and it was demonstrated that similar improvements were made in both groups. Other investigations of elderly men and women using systematic exercise programmes showed significant improvements in both upper and lower limb joints (Lesser 1978; Raab *et al.*, 1988) and in the thigh extensors and lower back (Frekany and Leslie, 1975).

IMPLICATIONS FOR RECREATIONAL ACTIVITY

Although adaptations are inevitable in the body tissues and systems as people age, it is evident that these changes are exacerbated by decreasing levels of regular physical activity. Sedentary people have a decreased functional capacity when compared with their more active peers and this leads to decrements in the performance of daily living activities. It has also been shown that increased activity produces adaptations favouring muscular strength and endurance. The important point is that older people do respond to physical training, and that all aspects of functional capacity studied have responded favourably to increased activity levels.

Therefore, as in the general population, the level of physical well-being of an adult with Down syndrome is an important factor in determining the functional impact of ageing changes. Janicki and Jacobsen (1986) have shown that functional capacities decline during the sixth decade in people with intellectual disabilities and this decline is reflected in the loss of skills in the fundamental activities of daily living. Also, the age-related decrease in physical endurance may limit leisure activities and community interactions, further restricting environmental stimulation so necessary to the quality of life. Another limiting factor in Down syndrome may be high obesity levels that affect the way a person performs activities, especially in terms of speed and energy costs.

There is evidence that people with intellectual disabilities can acquire basic recreation skills (Schloss *et al.*, 1986; King and Mace, 1990) and use community recreation and leisure activities. Appropriate leisure skills have been shown also to decrease inappropriate social and stereotypic behaviours (Schleien *et al.*, 1981). Yet at a time when an adequate level of activity is necessary, recreational participation is so often limited to non-participant activities such as watching television and listening to the radio (Schleien *et al.*, 1981).

Regular physical activity is important for older adults with Down syndrome in helping them to cope successfully with the demands of daily living and in the maintenance of social skills. There are many age-appropriate activities which can be incorporated into recreational and leisure programmes and which will provide these benefits.

Recreational activities

Walking is an ideal activity, and one which most older people find enjoyable, particularly if a walking track through a park can be used, or walking can be allied with another interest (Delehanty, 1985). Other physical activities which may be enjoyed by older people with Down syndrome include aerobics, weight lifting, hiking, and games such as bowls. With creative planning, it is possible to teach new sporting skills, including competitive play.

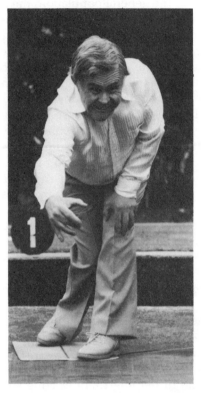

Figure 9.1 Outdoor bowling with friends (Reproduced with permission of the Australian Sport and Recreation Association for Persons with an Intellectual Disability.).

Swimming may also be popular with older people with Down syndrome in the future when the generations who have had swimming lessons during their school years grow older.

Swimming pool exercise such as 'aquarobics' which consists of walking with or without arm exercise has been suggested for older individuals with orthopaedic or other movement restriction (Claremont *et al.*, 1978). It has been shown that walking at thigh, waist, or chest immersion depth can promote a training effect, and so increase physical work

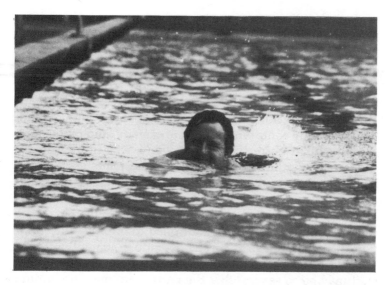

Figure 9.2 Swimming for enjoyment. (Reproduced with permission from Project Recreation, Ipswich, Queensland, Australia).

capacity. Calisthenics in a swimming pool may be used for muscle strengthening. The resistance and buoyancy of water enables many individuals to move muscles and joints in a less stressful way than may be possible out of the water. In general, water offers an excellent setting for group exercise because there is no danger of falling, and even those who have discomfort or instability in standing can often participate in the water (Delehanty, 1985).

Implementation

Guiding principles for conducting programmes for older adults include the provision of appropriate physical facilities. It is important to choose areas for organized activity where heat and noise factors can be regulated. Many older individuals cannot cope with high ambient temperatures and are more susceptible to heat stress than younger adults (Drinkwater and Horvath, 1979). Limitations of eyesight are common in the older age groups, and the nature of the activity must permit the wearing of glasses, and it must be remembered that many people with Down syndrome have auditory problems. Proper precautions for the safety and progress of the participants should be kept in mind, and the danger signals of overexertion monitored by the leader.

A medical evaluation of each participant should be made to indicate any contra-indications to exercise, and participants should obtain correctly designed and well-fitting jogging shoes. The condition of the muscles and joints of the lower limbs may be a limiting factor in the early stages, especially if the participant has not exercised for some time. Therefore, to avoid complications, a new activity should be started cautiously and be carefully controlled to improve the condition of the muscles exercised. If gradual adaptation is not allowed to take place, damage caused by an over-vigorous start may be so severe, that the participant may discontinue exercising.

Group activities are desirable as the chances of an individual participating regularly are far greater than otherwise. In addition, groups are important for maintaining social interaction skills. An ideal medium is an adapted aerobics class, as it has been shown that adults with Down syndrome are capable of participating and learning suitable exercises (King and Mace, 1990). These classes are an ideal way of providing exercises designed to improve the components of fundamental fitness, general endurance, specific muscular strength and endurance, and joint mobility. They also provide a very valuable adjunct to other motor activities such as walking or swimming.

Another important aspect of such classes is that they can offer variety within the class structure and so should encourage ongoing participation (James and Parker, 1989). One way in which variety is provided is through the use of music, which is important for motivation and it is also a group unifier (Carter, 1988).

The rationale for the design of general exercise programmes can be considered by analysing the different elements of an exercise programme and the reasons for their inclusion.

EXERCISE PROGRAMME DESIGN

An exercise programme is composed of four basic elements. A warm up period in preparation for more vigorous activity; a general endurance (aerobic) conditioning period during which continuous whole body rhythmic exercise is performed; a period during which exercises are performed to condition specific muscle groups; and a cool down period for the body to return to near normal resting levels.

The warm up

Pre-exercise warm up is necessary to allow for the adaptation of the cardiovascular-respiratory system and to reduce the potential for muscle and joint injury. Ten to fifteen minutes in older people eliminates or reduces an ischemic response (Barnard *et al.*, 1973). This warm up segment serves to increase muscle and joint temperatures and also results in decreased joint fluid viscosity and increased extensibility of connective tissue structures. It consequently reduces resistance to movement in joints and muscles and should thus aid the prevention of musculoskeletal injury. Care must be taken to ensure that the ankle joint is properly warmed up before lower limb movements requiring good dynamic balance are performed.

Activities in the warm up should be organized to provide a near continuous flow of exercises which begin at a low intensity and gradually become more vigorous. Activities for all parts of the body and involving all major joints should be included with a combination of rhythmical movements of gradually increasing range. It is ideal to begin with movements for which good adaptation has been preserved and then to have other movements organized so that the exercise sequence moves easily from one movement to another. Participants may be seated on chairs in a circle at the beginning of the programme and then move to a standing position. The warm up should conclude with chairs out of the way, and participants standing.

General endurance conditioning

The aerobic conditioning section which follows the warm up

should aim at relatively low intensity activity sustained over a period of no less than 15 minutes. A variety of rhythmic locomotor activities can be utilized, such as simple walking patterns combined with either free form arm movements, and some follow the leader movements. Stimulating music is the key, with well chosen rhythm which encourages people to move briskly.

The first activity can be a walk routine incorporating simple upper limb movements. This can be followed by a combination of walk and simple dance steps such as twisting. More advanced groups can also use dumb-bells in the hands to increase the intensity level of the walk routines. Simple walking can be used between the different segments. There should be some progression in the intensity level of the sequences, alternation between easier and more energetic sequences may be best, but this section must always conclude with a less vigorous sequence.

Good aerobic capacity is advantageous in everyday life in reducing the effort required to cope successfully with the demands of being relatively independent and mobile within the community. One practical aspect is that it is important to be able to walk fast and maintain a good balance for crossing a traffic-bearing street, or to be able to hurry to catch a bus or train.

Muscular conditioning

The emphasis should be placed on improving the strength and endurance of specific muscle groups, particularly those (a) directly responsible for everyday skills essential for independent self maintenance; (b) which provide for a good standing posture; and (c) which counteract the effects of habitual activities by trying to correct muscular strength imbalances in antagonistic muscle groups.

An important consideration in this part of the exercise programme is to create local muscular endurance which implies the ability to repeat the contraction of a single muscle group. It is therefore necessary to apply the principle of overload and maintain the work for the selected muscle group at a relatively high level, but without creating local fatigue. This may be achieved by moving from one exercise to another for a different muscle group. Also half the repetitions may be performed at one time, and the other half at another. Exercise should be organized in a progressive way, so that the difficulty, both in the strength required, and the co-ordination necessary, increases from week to week.

Bean bags are a valuable adjunct to strengthening exercises. They are most commonly held in the hand, and can be used to increase the intensity of exercises for the upper limb and shoulder girdle. Bean bags also aid in creating some variety in the programme and can be used for passing movements such as from one hand to another, or from one person to another. To serve the same purpose, dumb-bells can be used, and may appeal to men, because of the association with weight lifting. Some very imaginative ideas for exercise are available using coloured rubber bands. These are excellent for strengthening exercises as they are very versatile and can be used across the ankles or be held in the hands.

The primary muscle group to focus on in the lower limb is the quadriceps because of its role in important daily activities such as stair climbing, rising from chairs, and negotiating high steps in getting in and out of public transport. In addition, important postural muscles for attention are the plantar flexors of the foot and the hamstrings which help balance the trunk in concert with the gluteals, particularly in dynamic situations.

The intrinsic muscles of the feet should be exercised. The muscles under the foot atrophy with age, and as the fat pad also decreases, the bones have very little protection by way of the shock absorbing qualities offered by these tissues. Because we mostly wear shoes, and these hold toes in a relatively rigid position, the muscles receive little exercise in movements such as curling the toes. This exercise should be reserved for just prior to the cool down so that shoes may be removed. Examples include trying to pick up pencils or marbles from the floor, or moving forward with the toes working in a wormlike way to edge the body forward.

The choice of movements for the upper limbs and shoulder girdle should consider muscle activity in making use of the hands in dressing and housekeeping, transferring objects from one level to another, balancing via a firm hand grip, and using the arms for recruiting thrust when attempting to rise from a low chair. Exercise involving supination of the hand is important and the strength of the fingers should be maintained with activities such as squeezing a small rubber ball. The extensors of the elbow (triceps) are important for many skills, and exercises incorporating a modified push up against the wall or a chair seat could be used. This exercise would be valuable also for improving the pectoralis major muscle which is important in many housekeeping tasks.

Care is needed to avoid muscle imbalance so the muscles of the posterior shoulder girdle must not be neglected. In addition, these muscles help keep the shoulders correctly positioned. Other major postural muscle groups include the abdominals, spinal extensors and gluteals and warrant specific attention before the class participants become fatigued.

The abdominal musculature plays a role in the posture of the pelvis and of the vertebral column. Exercises which require greater involvement of the abdominals than of the hip flexors should be chosen, because of the tendency for a strength imbalance between these groups. Activity for the extensors of the trunk and neck is also very necessary for this age group.

Some of these exercises can be conducted from an all fours position, or with the hands on the seat of a chair with the trunk as horizontal as possible. This will provide work for the neck extensors, as the head is held in position against gravity while the participant looks towards the leader and at other class members. The gluteals can be exercised also from this position with movements involving one of the lower limbs. These muscles which are active in locomotion also help position the pelvis and decrease the tendency to a lordosis.

The cool down

The cool down period is an ideal time for joint mobility conditioning as the core temperature will still be high and temperature affects the mechanics of connective tissue (Lehmann *et al.*, 1974). Range of motion in most joints is limited primarily by one or more specialized connective tissue structures including tendons, ligaments, joint capsules and fascial sheaths. Although muscles are not predominantly connective tissue, the resistance to stretch in muscles is derived from the extensive connective tissue framework and sheathing within and around muscles, not from the myofibrillar elements.

This cool down part of the programme is executed very slowly and should be of at least ten minutes' duration to allow time for all important joint movements to be performed. The static stretching method should be used with movements performed very slowly, and the stretch held for a number of seconds. The majority of movements should be performed from a floor position, so that the movement can be done without concern for stability.

The choice of movements is very important, and consideration should be given to (a) maintaining the mobility necessary for everyday activities (b) counteracting the tendency to contracture by stretching joints in the planes of movement in which they are usually maintained in a restricted range, and (c) the mobility needs of the structures involved in achieving a good upright posture.

Joint movements for the lower limb should be those which take into account that sitting postures with flexed hips and knees maintain the iliopsoas, rectus femoris, hamstrings and the calf muscles in a shortened position. Adequate mobility in the hip flexors is necessary for a good posture of the pelvis, and contracture in this area has been noted in the general population (Stoudt, 1981; James and Parker, 1989). The hips of people with Down syndrome are generally hypermobile (James, 1983), and even though there may be reductions with age, more than adequate mobility may remain. Ankle mobility is important in stair climbing so dorsiflexion activities should not be overlooked.

Movements for shoulder mobility are required to maintain a good ability for reaching upwards, taking the hands above the head, comfortably combing or washing the hair, and coping with a clasp or zip at the back of the neck or behind the waist. Stretching of the anterior shoulder girdle is needed for a good postural alignment of the upper portion of the vertebral column. It will be necessary to offer stretching movements for the shoulders in all planes, as well as for the wrists, because their mobility is essential in everyday tasks. With regard to the trunk, mobility of the spine in forward flexion is perhaps the primary consideration in maintaining the ability to wash the feet, or put on stockings and shoes.

It is possible, however, that many people with Down syndrome will have adequate flexibility in this plane.

Compliance with an exercise programme

A problem with continued participation in activity programmes is sustaining the interest of participants. Many factors have been identified in motivating people to remain in exercise programmes, among which the most important undoubtedly are the ability and personality of the exercise leader and the composition of the programme.

There are a multitude of styles of leadership in keeping with the personality of the individual, however, there are certain traits necessary for the development of successful leadership. Above all, the leader must be enthusiastic, sensitive to the needs of the participants and to the physical limitations of this population. The ability to offer encouragement, even when minimal evidence of improvement is noted, is important.

Creativeness, interest and fun are necessary in preventing programmes from becoming boring. The use of music as a background to some endurance activities, or for exercises to be performed rhythmically enhances both mood and tolerance, and adds interest and variety to a programme. A variety of equipment can be used to make exercises more challenging and interesting.

A circular formation of chairs rather than the traditional lines should be explored for stationary exercises, so that all participants are able to see and hear the leader, and also have the opportunity to interact with others (Hansen, 1980). Size of the group is important, because too small a group may not encourage social interaction while too large a group may limit interpersonal relationships and make adequate supervision difficult.

AGEING, ACTIVITY, AND DOWN SYNDROME: EXTENDING THE CONTINUUM

The average lifespan for people with Down syndrome is longer than in the past, so that the proportion in the population who are elderly is rising. Many of these older adults with Down syndrome may be manifesting poorer function in social

skills, conversational ability, and coping with the fundamental activities of daily living than they need be because of
their lifestyle.

In the past, adults with Down syndrome received little in
the way of health education or training in such lifestyle factors
as nutrition and physical activity. They had a very limited and
sedentary repertoire of leisure skills (Cheseldine and Jeffree,
1981; Schleien *et al.*, 1981; Carter, 1988) and did not become
involved with adult physical activities, especially those that
fostered endurance. This pattern of reduced physical activity
could result in people showing functional impairment very
quickly when age-related changes begin, and so predispose
them to premature separation from community interaction by
reducing mobility and physical independence.

Major changes have taken place in social and educational
experiences over several decades and there is now an expectation that older people with Down syndrome will engage in
more active and varied leisure activities. In the absence of a
specific medical problem there is no reason why such people
should not lead full and active lives (Delehanty, 1985). Active
recreation provides not merely a way of filling in time but is
an important context in which social relationships are maintained.

There is a dearth of knowledge about many aspects of
ageing in Down syndrome, in particular, the timetable of
physiological events and the range of individual variation. This
is perhaps because only recently have persons with Down
syndrome begun to reach middle age as community residents
(Schleien *et al.*, 1981). This information is important for determining the functional impact of age changes. We need to know
when the decline begins, which functions are involved,
and how these decrements affect the performance of daily
living activities. At the functional level, the question of what
tasks people with Down syndrome need to perform on a
daily basis in order to maintain independence and a satisfactory quality of life requires further attention. Little is known
about how elderly persons with Down syndrome spend their
days, and even less is known about their personal satisfaction with their activities or inactivity (Seltzer, 1985). It is evident
that the process and consequences of ageing is an area that
warrants an increased research effort.

It should be possible to help people with Down syndrome maintain a focus on leisure and social interaction in the same way as their non-handicapped peers. Access to, and instruction in the use of different recreational activities, should be available at the different stages of adult life, so that adults with Down syndrome can enjoy the reinforcing aspects of physical activity. To do this, it is necessary that a focus on preventive health practices and maintenance of optimum physical function begin in adolescence, and that the activity skills taught are evaluated for their relevance to both enjoyment and function in adulthood. Because of the value of general conditioning programmes in maintaining both general and specific aspects of fitness, such programmes should figure highly in the physical education activities of older school children with Down syndrome.

The basic challenge which must be met for elderly people with Down syndrome, is how to extend and improve the quality of their lives. In order to provide effectively and creatively for their needs, the continuum of social, educational and recreational experiences begun in childhood should be extended to cover the full life cycle.

Appendix A: Glossary

Abduction: movement away from the midline of the body.

Adduction: movement towards the midline of the body.

Atlanto-axial joints: the joints between the atlas and the axis vertebrae. The atlas, carrying the skull, rotates on the axis at the atlanto-axial joints, pivoting on the dens (odontoid process).

Atlas: the first cervical vertebra.The skull rests on the atlas.

Axis (vertebra): the second cervical vertebra around which the atlas turns. The dens of odontoid process projects upwards and develops as the pivot for the atlas.

Dens or odontoid process: the part of the axis (vertebra) that projects upwards like a peg and on which the atlas pivots.

Dorsiflexion: bending of the foot upwards with toes pulled up towards knee (as in walking uphill).

Gluteal muscles: muscles controlling hip movement (gluteus maximus, gluteus medius, gluteus minimus).

Hypoplasia of the odontoid process: under-formation or developmental deficiency of the odontoid process (see dens).

Isokinetic strength: ability of the muscle to contract at a fixed speed against a variable resistance.

Isometric strength: muscular exercise in which the muscle contracts but movement is counteracted i.e. distance between body parts remains the same.

Joint subluxation: partial dislocation of joint.

Landau response: automatic postural reaction of extension of trunk and hips when baby is held in a horizontal position.

Pectoralis major muscle: a large chest muscle.

Plantarflexion: bending of the foot downwards (as in walking downhill).

Sarcomeres: a bundle of fibres within muscle cells that are responsible for contraction of the muscle.

Synovial joints: freely moveable joints with a cavity containing a fluid (synovia) that lubricates the joint (e.g. elbow).

References

Abroms, K. and Bennett, J. (1981) Parental contributions to Trisomy 21: Review of recent cytological and statistical findings, in *Frontiers of Knowledge in Mental Retardation, Vol. II* – Biomedical Aspects, (ed. P. Mittler), University Park Press, Baltimore, pp. 149–57.

Adams G.M. and de Vries, H.A. (1973) Physiological effects of an exercise training regimen upon women aged 52 to 79. *Journal of Gerontology*, **28**, 50–5.

Akeson, W.H., Amiel, D., Abel, M.F., Gardin, S.R. and Woo, S. L-Y (1987) Effects of immobilization on joints. *Clinical Orthopaedics*, 28–37.

Allander, E., Bjornsson, O.J., Olafsson, O., Sigfusson, N. and Thorsteinsson, J. (1974) Normal range of joint movements in shoulder, hip, wrist and thumb with special reference to side: a comparison between two populations. *International Journal of Epidemiology*, **3**, 253–61.

Allen, T.H., Andersen, E.C. and Langham, W.H. (1960) Total body potassium and gross body composition in relationship to age. *Journal of Gerontology*, **15**, 348–57.

Alvarez, N. and Rubin, L. (1986) Atlantoaxial instability in adults with Down syndrome: a clinical and radiological survey. *Applied Research in Mental Retardation*, **7** (1), 67–78.

Aniansson, A., Grimby, G., Hedberg, M. and Rundgren, A. (1980) Isometric and isokinetic quadriceps muscle strength in 70-year old men and women. *Scandinavian Journal of Rehabilitation Medicine*, **12**, 161–8.

Aniansson, A., Grimby, G., Hedberg, M., Rundgren, A. and Sperling, L. (1978) Muscle function in old age. *Acta Physiologica Scandinavia*, Suppl 6, 43–9.

Aniansson, A. and Gustafsson, E. (1981) Physical training in elderly men with special reference to quadriceps muscle strength and morphology. *Clinical Physiology*, **1**, 87–98.

Aniansson, A., Ljungberg, P., Rundgren, A. and Wetterqvist, H. (1984a) Effect of a training programme for pensioners on condition and muscular strength. *Archives Gerontology and Geriatrics*, **3**, 229–41.

Aniansson, A., Sperling, L., Rundgren, A. and Lehnberg, E. (1983) Muscle function in 75-year-old men and women a longitudinal study. *Scandinavian Journal of Rehabilitation Medicine* Suppl. 9, 92–102.

Aniansson, A., Zetterberg, C., Hedberg, M. and Henriksson, K.G. (1984b) Impaired muscle function with aging. *Clinical Orthopaedics,* **191,** 193–201.

Anwar, F. (1981) Motor function in Down's syndrome. *International Review of Research in Mental Retardation,* **10,** 107–38.

Anwar, F. (1983) Vision and kinaesthesis in motor movements, in *Advances in mental handicap research,* Vol. 2., (eds J. Hogg and P.J. Mittler), John Wiley, London, pp. 203–31.

Balkany, T.J., Downs, M.P., Jafek, B.W. and Krajicek, M.J. (1979) Hearing loss in Down's syndrome, a treatable handicap more common than is generally recognized. *Clinical pediatrics,* **18,** 116–18.

Barden, H.S. (1983) Growth and development of selected hard tissues in Down syndrome: a review. *Human Biology,* **55,** 539–76.

Barnard, R.J., Gardner, G.W., Diaco, N.V., MacAlpin, R.N. and Kattus, A. (1973) Cardiovascular responses to sudden strenuous exercise – heart, blood pressure, and ECG. *Journal of Applied Physiology,* **34,** 938–46.

Barnet, A.B., Ohlrich, E.S. and Shanks, B.L. (1971) EEG evoked responses to repetitive auditory stimulation in normal and Down's Syndrome infants. *Developmental Medicine and Child Neurology,* **13,** 321–9.

Bassey, E.J. (1978) Age, inactivity and some physiological responses to exercise. *Gerontology,* **24,** 66–77.

Beasley, C.R. (1982) Effects of a jogging program on cardiovascular fitness and work performance of mentally retarded adults. *American Journal of Mental Deficiency,* **86,** 609–13.

Beeghly, M., Weiss-Perry, B. and Cicchetti, D. (1989) Structural and affective dimensions of play development in young children with Down syndrome. *International Journal of Behavioral Development,* **12** (2), 257–7.

Bell, R.D. and Hoshizaki, T.B. (1981) Relationships of age and sex with range of motion of seventeen joint actions in humans. *Canadian Journal of Applied Sport Science,* **6,** 202–6.

Bennet, G.C., Rang, M., Roye, D.P. and Aprin, H. (1982) Dislocation of the hip in trisomy 21, *The Journal of Bone and Joint Surgery,* **64** (3), 289–94.

Bergen, D. (ed.) (1988) *Play as a Medium for Learning and Development. A Handbook of Theory and Practice,* Heinemann, New Hampshire.

Bergmann, K. (1990) Incidence of atypical pencil grasps among non-dysfunctional adults. *American Journal of Occupational Therapy,* **44,** 736–40.

Bergstrom, G., Aniansson, A., Belle, A. *et al.* (1985) *Scandinavian Journal of Rehabilitation Medicine,* **17,** 183–90.

Bobath, K. and Bobath, B. (1972) Diagnosis and assessment of cerebral palsy, in *Physical Therapy Services in the Developmental*

Disabilities, (eds P.H. Pearson and C.E. Williams), Charles C. Thomas, Springfield, Illinois, pp. 31–113.

Boone, D.C. and Azen, S.P. (1979) Normal joint of motion at joints in male subjects. *Journal of Bone and Joint Surgery*, **61-A**, 756–9.

Boone, D.C., Walker, J.M. and Perry, J. (1981) Age and sex differences in lower extremity joint motion. Abstract, *Physical Therapy*, **61**, 688.

Borkan, G.A. and Norris, A.H. (1977) Fat redistribution and the changing body dimensions of the adult male. *Human Biology*, **49**, 495.

Borkan, G.A., Hults, D.E., Gerzof, S.G. and Robbins, A.H. (1985) Comparison of body composition in middle-aged and elderly males using computed tomography. *American Journal of Physical Anthropology*, **66**, 289–95.

Brewer, N., Cunningham, S. and White, J.M. (1989/1990). A computerized procedure for teaching letter formation skills to mentally retarded individuals. *Journal of Educational Technology Systems*, **18**, 185–90.

Bronks, R. and Parker, A.W. (1985) Anthropometric observation of adults with Down syndrome. *American Journal of Mental Deficiency* **90** (1), 110–13.

Brooks, D.N., Wooley, H. and Kanjilal, G.C. (1972) Hearing loss and middle ear disorders in patients with Down's syndrome (mongolism). *Journal of Mental Deficiency Research*, **16**, 21–9.

Brown, J.K. (1974) General Neurology, in *Neonatal Medicine*, (eds F. Cockburn and C. Drillien), Blackwell Scientific Pub., Oxford, pp. 520–42.

Brown, M. (1987) Change in fibre size, not number, in ageing skeletal muscle. *Age and Ageing*, **16**, 244–8.

Brown, P. (1980) Fitness and Play, in *In Celebration of Play*, (ed. P.F. Wilkinson), Croom Helm, London, pp. 282–95.

Buckley, S. (1987) Attaining basic educational skills: reading, writing and number, in *Current Approaches to Down's Syndrome*, (eds D. Lane and B. Stratford), Cassell, London, pp. 315–43.

Bullough, P.G. (1981) The geometry of diarthrodial joints, its physiologic maintenance, and the possible significance of age-related changes in geometry-to-load distribution and the development of osteoarthritis. *Clinical Orthopaedics*, **156**, 61–6.

Burkhart, J.E., Fox, R.A. and Rotatori, A.F. (1985) Obesity of mentally retarded individuals: Prevalence, characteristics and intervention. *American Journal of Mental Deficiency*, **90** (3), 303–12.

Burnett, C.N. and Johnson E.W. (1971) Development of gait in childhood, Part ii. *Developmental Medicine and Child Neurology*, **13**, 207–15.

Burns, Y.R., Ensbey, R.M. and Norrie, M.A. (1989) The neurosensory motor developmental assessment Part i: Development and administration. *Australian Journal of Physiotherapy*, **35**, 141–9.

Butterworth, G. and Cicchetti, D. (1978) Visual calibration of posture in normal and motor retarded Down's syndrome infants. *Perception*, **7**, 513–25.

Butterworth, G. and Hicks, L. (1977) Visual proprioception and postural stability in infancy: A developmental study. *Perception*, **6**, 255–62.

Campbell, M.J., McComas, A.J. and Petito, F. (1973) Physiological changes in ageing muscles. *Journal of Neurology*, **36**, 174–82.

Carleton, N.L. (1989) Chute the works: motivating fitness and movement. *JOPERD*, **60** (1), 73–8.

Carter, J. (1988). *Creative day-care for mentally handicapped people*, Basil Blackwell, Oxford.

Carter, M. (1991) Getting to grips with handwriting. *Special Children*, 7–9.

Chad, K., Jobling, A. and Frail, H. (1990) Metabolic rate: A factor in developing obesity in children with Down syndrome? *American Journal of Mental Retardation*, **95** (2), 228–35.

Chapman, E., de Vries, H.A. and Swezey, R. (1972) Joint stiffness: effects of exercise on young and old men. *Journal of Gerontology*, **27**, 218–21.

Cheseldine, S.E. and Jeffree, D.M. (1981) Mentally handicapped adolescents: Their use of leisure. *Journal of Mental Deficiency Research*, **25**, 49–59.

Chumlea, W.C. and Baumgartner, R.N. (1989) Status of anthropometry and body composition data in elderly subjects. *American Journal of Clinical Nutrition*, **50**, 1158–66.

Cicchetti, D. and Sroufe, L. (1976) The relationship between affective and cognitive development in Down syndrome infants. *Child Development*, **47**, 920–29.

Claremont, A.D., Smith E. and Reddan, W. (1978) Swimming pool exercises for the aged. *Medicine and Science in Sports*, **10**, 55.

Clark, D.L., Kruetzberg, J.R. and Chee, F.K.W. (1977) Vestibular stimulation influence on motor development in infants. *Science*, **196**, 1228–9.

Clay, M. (1975) *What did I write?* Heinemann Educational, Auckland, N.Z.

Cody, K.A. and Nelson, A.J. (1978) The effect of verticality perception on body balance in normal subjects. *Physical Therapy*, **58**, 35–41.

Cole, D.A. (1986) Facilitating play in children's peer relationships: Are we having fun yet? *American Educational Research Journal*, **23** (2), 201–15.

Collette, M.A. (1979) Dyslexia and classic pathognomic signs. *Perceptual and Motor Skills*, **37**, 1055–62.

Committee on Sports Medicine. (1984) Atlantoaxial instability in Down syndrome. *Pediatrics*, **74** (1), 152–4.

Connolly, K., and Dalgleish, M. (1989) The emergence of a tool-using skill in infancy. *Developmental Psychology*, **25** (6), 894–912.

Copley, J. and Ziviani, J. (1990) Kinaesthetic sensitivity and handwriting ability in grade one children. *Australian Journal of Occupational Therapy*, **37**, 39–43.

Corbin C. and Lindsey, R. (1984) *The Ultimate Fitness Book: Physical Fitness Forever*, Leisure Press, New York.

Cowie, V. (1970) *A Study of the Early Development of Mongols,* Pergamon Press, Oxford.

Cranach, M. von (1982) The psychological study of goal-directed action: Basic issues, in *The Analysis of Action: Recent Theoretical and Empirical Advances* (eds M. von Cranach and R. Harre), Cambridge University Press, Cambridge, pp. 35–73.

Cratty, B.J. (1971) *Active Learning,* Prentice-Hall Inc., New Jersey.

Cratty, B.J. (1974) *Motor activity and the education of retardates,* Lea & Febiger, Philadelphia.

Cratty, B.J. (1979) *Perceptual and Motor Development in Infants and Children,* 2nd edn, Prentice-Hall Inc., New Jersey.

Crombie, M., Gunn, P. and Hayes, A. (1991) A longitudinal study of two cohorts of children with Down syndrome, in *Adolescents with Down syndrome: International perspectives on research and programme development,* (ed. C.J. Denholm), University of Victoria, Victoria, Canada, pp. 3–14.

Cronk, C.F., Chumlea, W.C., and Roche, A.F. (1985) Assessment of overweight children with trisomy 21. *American Journal of Mental Deficiency,* **89** (4), 433–6.

Csikszentmihalyi, M. (1975) *Beyond Boredom and Anxiety,* Jossey-Bass Publishers, London.

Cunningham, C.C. (1982) *Down's Syndrome: An Introduction for Parents,* Souvenir Press, London.

Cunningham, C.C. and Glenn, S.M. (1987) Parent involvement and early intervention, in *Current Approaches to Down's Syndrome* (eds D. Lane and B. Stratford), Cassell, Gillingham, Kent, pp. 347–62.

Cunningham, C.C., Glenn, S.M., Wilkinson, P. and Sloper, P. (1984) Mental ability, symbolic play and receptive and expressive language of young children with Down syndrome. *Journal of Child Psychology,* **26** (2) 255–65.

Cunningham, D.A., Morrison, D., Rice, C.L. and Cooke, C. (1987) Ageing and isokinetic plantar flexion. *European Journal of Applied Physiology,* **56**, 24–39.

Dahle, A.J., and McCollister, F.P. (1986) Hearing and otologic disorders in children with Down's Sydnrome. *American Journal of Mental Deficiency,* **90** (60), 636–42.

Dalgleish, M. (1977) *The Development of Tool Using Skills in Infancy,* Unpublished doctoral dissertation, University of Sheffield, Sheffield.

Damon, A., Seltzer, C.C., Stoudt, H.W. and Bell, B. (1972) Age and physique in healthy white veterans. *Journal of Gerontology,* **27**, 202–8.

Danneskiold-Samsoe, B., Kofod, V., Munter, J. *et al.* (1984) Muscle strength and functional capacity in 78–81-year-old men and women. *European Journal of Applied Physiology,* **52**, 310–14.

Davis, W.E. (1986) Development of control and co-ordination in the mentally handicapped, in *Themes in Motor Development,* (eds H.T.A. Whiting and M.G. Wade), Martinus Nijhoff Publishers, Dordrecht, The Netherlands, pp. 143–58.

Davis, W.E. and Kelso, J.A.S. (1982) Analysis of 'invariant characteristics' in the motor control of Down's syndrome and normal subjects. *Journal of Motor Behaviour*, **14**, 194–212.

Davis, W.E. and Sinning, W.E. (1987) Muscle stiffness in Down syndrome and other mentally handicapped subjects: A research note. *Journal of Motor Behavior*, **19** (1), 130–44.

Delehanty, M.J. (1985) Health care and inhome environments, in *Aging and Developmental Disabilities*, (eds M.P. Janecki and H.M. Wisniewski), Paul H. Brookes, Baltimore, pp. 211–323.

Dequeker, J., Goris, P. and Uytterhoeven, R. (1983) Osteoporosis and osteoarthritis (osteoarthrosis). *JAMA*, **249**, 1448–51.

de Vries, J.P., Visser, G.H.A. and Prechtl, H.F.R. (1985) The emergence of fetal behaviour, 11: Quantitative aspects. *Early Human Development*, **12**, 99–120.

Diamond, L.S., Lynne, D. and Sigman, B. (1981) Orthopedic disorders in patients with Down's Syndrome. *Orthopedic Clinics of North America*, **12** (1), 57–71.

Dienes, Z.P. (1973) *Mathematics through the Senses, Games, Dance and Arts*, NFER, Windsor, Berks.

DiRocco, P.J., Clarke, J.E. and Phillips, S.J. (1987) Jumping co-ordination patterns of mildly mentally retarded children. *Adapted Physical Activity Quarterly*, **4**, 178–91.

Down, J.L.H. (1866) Some observations on an ethnic classification of idiots. *Clinical Lectures and Reports*, London Hospital, **3**, 259.

Drinkwater, B.L. and Horvath, S.M. (1979) Heat tolerance and aging. *Medicine and Science in Sports*, **11**, 49–55.

Dubowitz, V. (1980) *The floppy infant* 2nd edn, Clinics in Developmental Medicine No. 76, Spastics International Publications, Heinemann, London.

Duffy, L. and Wishart, J.G. (1987) A comparison of two procedures for teaching discrimination skills to Down Syndrome and non-handicapped children. *British Journal of Educational Psychology*, **57** (3), 265–78.

Dupont, A., Vaeth, M. and Videbech, P. (1986) Mortality and life expectancy in Down's syndrome in Denmark. *Journal of Mental Deficiency Research*, **30**, 111–20.

Dyer, S. and Berry, P. (1991) A health-related fitness programme for adolescents with Down syndrome: A single case study, in *Adolescents with Down Syndrome: International Perspectives on Research and Programme Development*, (ed. C.J. Denholm), University of Victoria, Victoria, Canada, pp. 159–74.

Dyer, S., Gunn, P., Rauh, H. and Berry, P. (1990) Motor development in Down syndrome children. An analysis of the motor scale of the Bayley Scales of Infant Development, in *Motor development, adapted physical activity and mental retardation*, (ed. A. Vermeer), Karger, Basel, pp. 7–20.

Elliott, D. (1990) Movement control and Down syndrome: A neuro-psychological approach, in *Problems in Movement Control*, (ed. G. Reid), Elsevier Science, Amsterdam, N.H, pp. 201–16.

Elliott, D., Weeks, D.J. and Elliott, C.L. (1987) Cerebral specialization in individuals with Down Syndrome. *American Journal on Mental Retardation*, **92** (3), 263–71.

Ellis, M.J. and Scholtz, G.J.L. (1978) *Activity and Play of Children*, Prentice-Hall, Englewood Cliffs, New Jersey.

Emes, C., Velde, B., Moreau, M., Murdoch, D.D. and Trussell, R. (1990) An activity based weight control program. *Adapted Phyiscal Activity Quarterly*, **7**, 314–24.

Erhardt, R.P. (1974) Sequential levels in development of prehension. *American Journal of Occupational Therapy*, **28**, 592–6.

Espenschade, A.S. and Eckert, H.M. (1980) *Motor Development*, 2nd edn, Charles E. Merrill and Bell and Howell, Columbus, Ohio.

Essen-Gustavsson, B. and Borges, O. (1986) Histochemical and metabolic characteristics of human skeletal muscle in relation to age. *Acta Physiologica Scandinavia*, **126**, 107–14.

Eyman, R. K., Call, T.L. and White, J.F. (1991) Life expectancy of persons with Down syndrome. *American Journal on Mental Retardation*, **95** (6), 603–12.

Feuerstein, R., Rand, Y. and Rynders, J.E. (1988) *Don't accept me as I am: Helping 'retarded' people to excel*, Plenum Press, New York.

Fiorentino M. (1972) *Normal and Abnormal Development: The Influence of Primitive Reflexes on Motor Development*, Charles C. Thomas, Springfield, Illinois.

Flavell, J.H. (1963) *The Developmental Psychology of Jean Piaget*, Van Nostrand, Princeton, N.J.

Forbes, G. (1976) The adult decline in lean body mass. *Human Biology*, **48**, 161–73.

Fort, P., Lifshitz, F., Bellisario, R., Davis, J., Lanes, R., Pugliese, M., Richman, R., Post, E.M. and David, R. (1984) Abnormalities of thyroid function in infants with Down syndrome. *The Journal of Pediatrics*, **104**, 545–9.

Fowler, J.S. (1981) *Movement Education*, Saunders College Publishing, Philadelphia.

Freeman, J.M. and Brann, A.W. (1977) Central Nervous System Disturbances, in *Neonatal-Perinatal Medicine* 2nd edn (ed. R.E. Behrman), C.V. Mosby Co., St Louis.

Freeman, J.M. and Myer, E.C. (1973) Central Nervous System Disturbances, in *Neonatology*, (ed. R.E. Behrman), C.V. Mosby Co., St Louis, pp. 517–62.

Frekany, G.A. and Leslie, D.K. (1975) Effects of an exercise program on selected flexibility measurements of senior citizens. *Gerontologist*, **15**, 182–8.

Froklis, V.V., Martynenko, O.A. and Zamostyan, V.P. (1976) Aging of the neuromuscular apparatus. *Gerontology*, **22**, 244–79.

Fryers, T. (1986) Survival in Down's syndrome. *Journal of Mental Deficiency Research*, **30**, 101–10.

Glean, G.P. van, Meulenbroek, R.G.J. and Hylkema, H.I. (1986) On the simultaneous processing of words, letters and strokes in handwriting. Evidence for a mixed linear and parallel model, in

Graphonomics: Contemporary Research in Handwriting, (eds H.S.R. Kao, G.P. van Galen and R. Hoosain), Amsterdam, North Holland.

Gallahue, D.L. (1989) *Understanding Motor Development. Infants, Children and Adults*, Benchmark Press Inc, Indianapolis, Indiana.

Gallahue, D.L., Werner, P.H. and Leudke, G.C. (1975) *A conceptual approach to moving and learning*, John Wiley, New York.

Gibson, D. (1989) The potential of syndrome-specific research for more effective assessment and psycho-educational intervention. *European Journal of Psychology and Education*, **4** (2), 247–9.

Gibson, D. (1991) Searching for a life-span psychobiology of Down syndrome: Advancing educational and behavioural management strategies. *International Journal of Disability, Development and Education*, **38** (1), 71–89.

Gibson, D. and Fields, D.L. (1984) Early infant stimulation programs for children with Downs Syndrome: A review of effectiveness. *Advances in Developmental and Behavioural Pediatrics*, **5**, 331–71.

Gibson, D. and Harris, A. (1988) Aggregated early intervention effects for Down's Syndrome persons: patterning and longevity of benefits. *Journal of Mental Deficiency Research*, **32**, 1–17.

Giebink, G.S. and Daly, K. (1990) Epidemiology and management of otitis media in children. *Topics in Language Disorders*, **11** (1), 1–10.

Ginn, E. (1988) *Critical power: A method for determination of the upper limit of aerobic capacity*, Unpublished thesis, University of Queensland.

Goodkin, F. (1980) The development of mature patterns of head-eye co-ordination in the human infant. *Early Human Development*, **4**, 373–87.

Goodnow, J. (1977) *Children drawing*, Harvard University Press, Cambridge, Mass.

Gould, D. (1984) Psychosocial development and children's sport, in *Motor Development during Childhood and Adolescence*, (ed. J.R. Thomas), Burgess Publishing, Minnesota, pp. 212–36.

Groner, Y., Dafni, M., Sherman, L., Levanon, D., Bernstein, Y., Danciger, E., Elroy-Stein, O. and Neer, A. (1986) Down's syndrome and Alzheimer's disease: Are common genes from human chromosome 21 involved in both disorders? in *Advances in Human Biology Vol. 29*, (eds A. Fisher, I. Hannin and C. Lachman), Plenum Press, New York, pp. 271–85.

Gunn, P. (1987) Speech and language, in *Current Approaches to Down's Syndrome*, (eds D. Lane and B. Stratford), Cassell, London, pp. 260–81.

Gunn, P. and Berry, P. (1985) Down's syndrome temperament and maternal response to descriptions of child behavior. *Developmental Psychology*, **21** (5), 842–47.

Gunn, P., and Berry, P. (1989) Education of infants with Down syndrome. *European Journal of Psychology of Education*, **4** (2), 235–46.

Gunn, P. and Cuskelly, M. (1991) Down syndrome temperament: The stereotype at middle childhood and adolescence. *International Journal of Disability, Development and Education*, **38** (1), 59–70.

Gunn, P., Berry, P. and Andrews, R.J. (1982) Looking behavior of Down syndrome infants. *American Journal of Mental Deficiency*, **87**, 344–7.

Guralnick, M.J. (1990) Major Accomplishment and future directions in early childhood mainstreaming. *Topics in Early Childhood Special Education*, **10** (2), 1–17.

Guralnick, M.J. and Groom, J.M. (1985) Correlates of peer-related social competence of developmentally delayed preschool children. *American Journal of Mental Deficiency*, **90** (2), 140–50.

Guralnick, M.J. and Groom, J.M. (1988) Friendships of preschool children in mainstreamed playgroups. *Developmental Psychology*, **24** (4), 595–604.

Guralnick, M.J. and Weinhouse, E. (1984) Peer-related social interactions of developmentally delayed young children: Development and characteristics. *Developmental Psychology*, **20** (5), 815–27.

Gutmann, E. and Hanzlikova, V. (1976) Fast and slow motor units in ageing. *Gerontology*, **22**, 280–300.

Hackett, L.C. (1970) *Movement exploration and games for the mentally retarded*, Peek Publications, Palo Alto, California.

Halar, E.M., Stolov, W.C., Venkatesh, B., Brozovich, F.V. and Harley, J.D. (1978) Gastrocnemius muscle belly and tendon length in stroke patients and able-bodied persons. *Archives of Physical Medicine and Rehabilitation*, **59**, 476–87.

Haley, S.M. (1986) Postural reactions in infants with Down syndrome: Relationship to motor milestone development and age. *Physical Therapy*, **66**, 17–22.

Haley, S.M. (1987) Sequence of development of postural reactions by infants with Down syndrome. *Developmental Medicine and Child Neurology*, **29**, 674–9.

Hall, D.A. (1976) *The aging of connective tissue*, Academic Press, New York.

Hallidie-Smith, K.A. (1987) The heart, in *Current Approaches to Down's Syndrome*, (eds D. Lane and B. Stratford), Cassell, Gillingham, Kent, pp. 53–70.

Hansen, J. (1980) Conditioning and aerobics for older Americans. *JOHPER*, **51** (2), 20–21.

Harris, S.R. (1980) Trans disciplinary model for the infant with Down's Syndrome. *Physical Therapy*, **60**, 420–23.

Harris, S.R. (1981) Effects of neurodevelopmental therapy on motor performance of infants with Down's Syndrome. *Developmental Medicine and Child Neurology*, **23**, 477–83.

Harris, S.R. (1984) Down Syndrome, in *Pediatric Neurologic Physical Therapy* (ed. S.K. Campbell), Churchill Livingstone, New York, pp. 169–204.

Harris, S.R. (1988) *Down's Syndrome: Papers and Abstracts for Professionals*, vol 11, no. 7, 1–4.

Hartley, X.Y. (1986) A summary of recent research into the development of children with Down's syndrome. *Journal of Mental Deficiency Research*, **30** (1), 1–14.

Haubenstricker, J., Branta, C. and Seefeldt, V. (1983) *Preliminary validation of developmental sequences for throwing and catching*, Paper presented at the Annual Conference of the North American Society for the Psychology of Sport and Physical Activity, East Lansing, Michigan.

Hayden, A.H. and Haring, N.G. (1978) Early intervention for high risk infants and young children: Programs for Down's syndrome children, in *Intervention strategies for high risk infants and young children*, (ed. T.D. Tjossem), University Park Press, Baltimore, pp. 573–608.

Hayes, A. and Gunn, P. (1991) Developmental assumptions about Down syndrome and the myth of uniformity, in *Adolescents with Down Syndrome: International Perspectives on Research and Programme Development*, (ed. C.J. Denholm), University of Victoria, Victoria, Canada, pp. 73–82.

Hemmert, T.J. (1979) An investigation of basic gross motor skill development of moderately retarded children and youth. *Dissertation Abstracts International*, **39**, 4807A.

Henderson, S.E. (1987) Motor skill development, in *Current Approaches to Down's Syndrome*, (eds D. Lane and B. Stratford), Cassell, Gillingham, Kent, pp. 187–218.

Hewitt, K.E. and Jancar, J. (1986) Psychological and clinical aspects of aging in Down syndrome, in *Science and service in mental retardation*, (ed. J.M. Berg), Paul H. Brookes, Baltimore, pp. 370–79.

Hewitt, K.E., Carter, G. and Jancar, J. (1985) Aging in Down's syndrome. *British Journal of Psychology*, **147**, 58–62.

Hofsten, C. von (1989) Motor development as the development of systems: comments on the special section. *Developmental Psychology*, **6**, 950–53.

Hogg, J. and Moss, S.C. (1983) Prehensile development in Down's syndrome and non-handicapped preschool children. *British Journal of Developmental Psychology*, **1**, 189–204.

Hogg, J. (1981) Learning, using and generalizing manipulative skills in a preschool classroom by nonhandicapped and Down's syndrome children. *Educational Psychology*, **1** (4), 319–40.

Hogg, J. (1986) Process and context in ensuring competent motor behavior by mentally retarded people, in *Motor Skill Acquisition of the Mentally Handicapped: Issues in Research and Training*, (ed. M.G. Wade), Elsevier Science, North Holland, pp. 227–41.

Holland, B.V. (1987) Fundamental motor skill performance of non-handicapped and educable mentally impaired students. *Education and Training in Mental Retardation*, **22** (3), 197–204.

Holle, B. (1976) *Motor Development in Children: Normal and Retarded*, Blackwell Scientific Publications, Oxford.

Holt, K.S. (1977) *Developmental Paedicatrics*, Postgraduate Paediatrics Series Butterworths, London and Boston.

Horgan, J.S. (1980) Pursuit rotor learning of mildly retarded children under supplementary feedback conditions. *Perceptual and Motor Skills*, **50**, 1219–28.

Howard, W.D. (1985) Atlanto-axial instability in Down syndrome: a need for awareness. *Mental Retardation,* **23** (4), 197–9.

Howe, B.L. (1988) Play and playfulness in physical education. *CAPHER Journal,* **54** (2), 6–9.

Hughes, N.A. (1971) Developmental Physiotherapy for mentally handicapped babies. *Physiotherapy,* **57**, 399–406.

Hunt, N. (1966) *The World of Nigel Hunt,* Darwen Finlayson, London.

Huson, A. (1984) Mechanics of joints. *International Journal of Sports Medicine,* **5**, 83–7.

Irwin, K.C. (1989) The school achievement of children with Down's syndrome. *New Zealand Medical Journal,* **102**, 11–13.

Jagjivan, B., Spencer, P.A. and Hosking, G. (1988) Radiological screening for atlanto-axial instability in Down's syndrome. *Clinical Radiology,* **39** (6), 661–3.

James, B. (1983) *Flexibility of Down Syndrome boys and girls,* Unpublished Thesis, Unviersity of Queensland.

James, B. (1991) *Locomotor function in elderly men and women,* Unpublished Thesis, University of Queensland.

James, B. and Parker, A.W. (1989) Active and passive mobility of lower limb joints in elderly men and women. *American Journal of Physical Medicine and Rehabilitation,* **68**, 252–8.

Janicki, M.P. and Jacobsen, J.W. (1986) Generational trends in sensory, physical and behavioral abilities among older mentally retarded persons. *American Journal of Mental Deficiency,* **90**, 490–500.

Johns, R.J. and Wright, V. (1962) Relative importance of various tissues in joint stiffness. *Journal of Applied Physiology,* **17**, 824–8.

Johnson, V. and Werner, R. (1980) *A Step by Step Learning Guide for Older Retarded Children,* Constable, London.

Jones, C. (1987) Using the soft-play room as an educational environment for young children and those with special educational needs. *British Journal of Physical Education,* **18** (5), 227–9.

Kaplan, F.S., Nixon, J.E., Reitz, M., Rindfleish, L. and Tucker, J. (1985) Age-related changes in proprioception and sensation in joint position. *Acta Orthopaedica Scandinavia,* **56**, 72–4.

Kasari, C., Mundy, P., Yirmiya, N. and Sigman, M. (1990) Affect and attention in children with Downs syndrome. *American Journal of Mental Deficiency,* **95** (1), 55–67.

Katz, R.C. and Singh, N.N. (1986) Increasing recreational behavior in mentally retarded children. *Behavior Modification,* **10**, 508–19.

Keiser, H. *et al.* (1981) Hearing loss of Downs Syndrome adults. *American Journal of Mental Deficiency,* **85** (5), 467–72.

Kelly, L.E., Rimmer, J.H. and Ness, R.A. (1986) Obesity levels in institutionalized mentally retarded adults. *Adapted Physical Activity Quarterly,* **3**, 167–76.

Kerr, B.A., McKerracher, D.W. and Neufeld, M. (1973) Motor assessment of the developmentally handicapped. *Perceptual and Motor Skills,* **36**, 139–46.

Kerr, R. and Blais, C. (1988) Directional probability information and

Down syndrome: A training study. *American Journal of Mental Retardation*, **92** (6), 531–8.

King, D. and Mace, F.C. (1990) Acquisition and Maintenance of Exercise Skills under Normalized Conditions by Adults with Moderate and Severe Mental Retardation. *Mental Retardation*, **28**, 311–17.

Kokmen, E., Bossemeyer, R.M., Barney, J. and Williams, R.J. (1977) Neurological manifestations of aging. *Journal of Gerontology*, **32**, 411–19.

Kovanen, V. (1989) Effects of ageing and physical training on rat skeletal msucle. *Acta Physiologica Scandinavia*, **Suppl. 135**, 1–56.

Krakow, J.B., and Kopp, C.B. (1982) Sustained attention in young Down syndrome children. *Topics in Early Childhood Special Education*, **2** (2), 32–42.

Kroll, W. and Clarkson, P.M. (1978) Age, isometric knee extension strength, and fractionated resisted response time. *Exp. Aging Research*, **4**, 389–409.

Krzywicki, H.J. and Chinn, K.S.K. (1967) Human body density and fat of an adult male population as measured by water displacement. *American Journal of Clinical Nutrition*, **20**, 305–310.

Kuta, I., Parizkova, J. and Dycka, J. (1970) Muscle strength and lean body mass in old men of different physical activity. *Journal of Applied Physiology*, **29**, 168–71.

Laban, R. (1956) *Principles of Dance and Movement Notation*, Macdonald and Evans, London

Laban, R. (1963) *Modern Educational Dance*, 2nd edition revised by L. Ullman, Praeger, New York.

Laban, R. (1971) *Mastery of Movement*, 3rd edtion revised by L. Ullman, MacDonald and Evans, London.

Lally, M. (1982) Computer-assisted handwriting instruction and visual/kinaesthetic feedback processes. *Applied Reserach in Mental Retardation*, **3**, 397–405.

Landry, S.H. and Chapieski, M.L. (1990) Joint attention of six-month old Down syndrome and preterm infants: 1. Attention to toys and mother. *American Journal on Mental Retardation*, **94** (5), 488–98.

Langendorfer, S. (1985) Label motor patterns, not kids: A developmental perspective for adapted physical education. *Physical Educator*, **42** (4), 175–9.

Larsson, L., Grimby, G. and Karlsson, J. (1979) Muscle strength and speed of movement in relation to age and muscle morphology. *Journal of Applied Physiology*, **46**, 451–6.

Larsson, L. and Karlsson, J. (1978) Isometric and dynamic endurance as a function of age and skeletal muscle characteristics. *Acta Physiologica Scandinava*, **104**, 129–36.

Lascelles, R.G. and Thomas, P.K. (1966) Changes due to age in internodal length in the sural nerve in man. *Journal of Neurology, Neurosurgery and Psychiatry*, **29**, 40–44.

Laszlo, J.I. and Bairstow, P.J. (1985). *Perceptual-motor behaviour: Development and therapy*, Holt Saunders, London.

Laszlo, J.I. and Broderick, P. (1991) Drawing and handwriting difficulties: Reasons for and remediation of dysfunction, in *Development of Graphic Skills*, (eds J. Wann, A.M. Wing and N. Sovik), Academic Press, London, pp. 259–80.

Laszlo, J.I. (1990). Child perceptuo-motor development: Normal and abnormal development of skilled behaviour, in *Developmental Psychology: Cognitive, Perceptuo-motor and Neurophysiological Perspective*, (ed. C.A. Hauert), Amsterdam, North Holland, pp. 273–308.

Lehmann , J.F., Ko, M.J. and deLateur, B.J. (1982) Knee movements; origin in normal ambulation and their modification by double stopped ankle-foot orthoses. *Archives Physical Medicine and Rehabilitation*, **63**, 345–51.

Leighton, J.R. (1957) Flexibility characteristics of four specialized skill groups of college athletes. *Archives of Physical Medicine and Rehabilitation*, **38**, 24–8.

Lejeune, J., Gautier, M. and Turpin, R. (1959) Etudes des chromosomes somatiques de neuf enfants mongoliens. *Comptes Rendues Academies Sciences (Paris)*, **248**, 1721–2.

Lesser, M. (1978) The effects of rhythmic exericse on the range of motion in older adults. *American Corrective Therapy Journal*, **32**, 118–22.

Levine, H.G. and Langness, L.L. (1983) Context, ability and performance: Comparison of competitive athletics among mildly mentally retarded and non-retarded adults. *American Journal of Mental Deficiency*, **87** (5), 528–38.

Lexell, J., Henriksson-Larsson, K., Winblad, B. and Sjostrom, M. (1983) Distribution of different fibre types in human skeletal muscle. 3. Effects of ageing on m. vastus lateralis studied in whole muscle cross-sections. *Muscle and Nerve*, **6**, 588–95.

Li, A.K.F. (1981). Play and the mentally retarded child. *Mental Retardation*, **19** (3), 121–6.

Libb, J.W., Myers, G.J., Graham, E. and Bell, B. (1985) Hearing disorder and cognitive function of individuals with Down syndrome. *American Journal of Mental Deficiency*, **90** (3), 353–6.

Lincoln, A.M., Courchesne, D., Kilman, B.A. and Galambos, R. (1985) Neuropsychological correlates of information-processing by children with Down syndrome. *American Journal of Mental Deficiency*, **89** (4), 403–14.

Lindboe, C.F. and Torvik, A. (1982) The effects of ageing, cachexia and neoplasms on striated muscle. *Acta Neuropathologica*, **57**, 85–92.

Linford, A.G., Jeanrenaud, C.Y., Karlson, K.A., Witt, P. and Linford, M.D. (1971) A computerized analysis of characteristics of Down's syndrome and normal children's free play. *Journal of Leisure Research*, **3** (1), 44–52.

Linford, A.G. and Duthie, J.H. (1970) The use of operant technology to induce sustained exertion in young trainable Down's syndrome children, in *Contemporary Sports Psychology*, (ed. G. Kenyon), The Athletic Institute, Chicago, 515–21.

Loovis, M.E. (1989) Climbing behavior of mentally retarded children: Developmental and environmental issues. *Physical Educator*, **46** (3), 149–53.

Lydic, J.S. and Steele, C. (1979) Assessment of the quality of sitting and gait patterns in children with Down's Synrome. *Physical Therapy*, **59**, 1489–94.

Lyons, M. (1986) Unlocking the closed doors of play. *Australian and New Zealand Journal of Developmental Disabilities*, **12** (4), 229–33.

Lyons, M. (1987) A Taxonomy of Playfulness for use in Occupational Therapy. *Australian Occupational Therapy Journal* **34** (4), 152–6.

MacTurk, R., Vietze, P., McCarthy, M., McQuiston, S. and Yarrow, L. (1985) The organization of exploratory behavior in Down syndrome and non-delayed infants. *Child Development*, **56**, 573–87.

Mahan, K.T., Diamond, E. and Brown, D. (1983) Podiatric profile of the Down's syndrome individual. *Journal of American Podiatry Association*, **73**, 173–8.

Malone, Q. (1988) Mortality and survival of the Down's syndrome population in Western Australia. *Journal of Mental Deficiency Research*, **32**, 59–65.

Masaki, M., Higurashi, M., Iijama, K. *et al.* (1981) Mortality and survival for Down's syndrome in Japan. *American Journal of Human Genetics*, **33**, 629–39.

McConkey, R. (1980) Designing and evaluating toys for the mentally handicapped child. *Journal of Practical Applications in Developmental Handicap*, **3**, 10–15.

McConkey, R. (1987) Play, in *Current approaches to Down syndrome*, (eds. D. Land and B. Stratford), Cassell, Gillingham, Kent, pp. 282–314.

McConkey, R. and Martin, H. (1983) Mothers' play with toys: a longitudinal study with Down's syndrome infants. *Child Care, Health and Development*, **9** (4), 215–26.

McConkey, R., Walsh, J. and Mulcahy, M. (1981) The recreational pursuits of mentally handicapped adults. *International Journal of Rehabilitation Research*, **4** (4), 493–9.

McDade, H. and Adler, S. (1980) Down Syndrome and short term memory impairment: A storage or not of retrieval deficit. *American Journal of Mental Deficiency*, **84**, 561–7.

McEnvoy, J. and McConkey, R. (1983) Play activities of mentally handicapped children at home and mothers' perceptions of play. *International Journal of Rehabiliation Research*, **6** (2), 143–51.

McKerracher, D.W. (1984) Progress in the assessment and prediction of vocational competence in the retarded, in *Integrated Programs for Handicapped Adolescents and Adults*, (ed. R.I. Brown), Croom Helm, London, pp. 23–60.

Meyers, L. (1988) Using computers to teach children with Down syndrome spoken and written language skills, in *Psychobiology of Down Syndrome*, (ed. L. Nadel), MIT Press, Boston, pp. 247–65.

Meyers, L. (1990) Language development and intervention, in *Clinical perspectives in the management of Down syndrome*, (eds C. van Dyke, D.C. Lang, F. Heide, S. van Dyke and M.J. Sovcek), Springer-Verlag, New York.

Miller, J. (1987) Language and communication characteristics of children with Down syndrome, in *New Perspectives on Down* syndrome (eds S. Pueschel *et al.*), Paul H. Brookes Publishing Co., Baltimore, pp. 233–62.

Miller, J. (1988) Developmental asynchrony of language development in children with Down syndrome, in *Psychobiology of Down Syndrome*, (ed. L. Nadel), MIT Press, Boston, pp. 167–98.

Miniszek, N.A. (1983) Development of Alzeheimer disease in Down Syndrome individuals. *American Journal of Mental Deficiency*, **87**, 377–85.

Miranda, S.B. and Fantz, R.L. (1973) Visual preferences of Down's syndrome and normal infants. *Child Development*, **44** (3), 555–61.

Miranda, S.B. and Fantz, R.L. (1974) Visual preferences of Down's syndrome and normal infants. *Child Development*, **44**, 555–61.

Mitchell, D.R. (1979) Parents as teachers of the handicapped. *Australian Journal of Physiotherapy, Paediatric Monograph*, 3–11.

Mojet, J. (1991) Characteristics of the developing handwriting skill in elementary education, in *Development of graphic skills*, (eds J. Wann, A.M. Wing and N. Sovik), Academic Press, London, pp. 53–74.

Morison, R. (1969) *A movement approach to educational gymnastics*, Bent and Sons, London.

Moritani, T. and de Vries, H.A. (1980) Potential for gross muscle hypertrophy in older men. *Journal of Gerontology*, **35**, 872–82.

Morris, A.F., Vaughn, S.E. and Vaccaro, P. (1982) Measurements of neuromuscular tone and strength in Down's syndrome children. *Journal of Mental Deficiency Research*, **26** (1), 41–6.

Moss, S.C. and Hogg, J. (1983) The development and integration of fine motor sequences in 12 to 18 month old children: A test of the modular theory of motor skill acquisition. *Genetic Psychology*, **107**, 145–87.

Mulholland, R. and McNeill, A.W. (1985) Cardiovascular responses of three profoundly retarded multiply handicapped children during selected motor activities, *Adapted Physical Activity Quarterly*, **2**, 151–60.

Mundy, P., Sigman, M., Kasari, C. and Yirmiya, N. (1988) Nonverbal communication skills in Down Syndrome children, *Child Development*, **59** (1), 235–49.

Murray, M.P., Gardner, G.M., Mollinger, L.A. and Sepic, S.B. (1980) Strength of isometric and isokinetic contractions. Knee muscles of men aged 20 to 86. *Physical Therapy*, **60**, 412–19.

Murray, M.P., Kory, R.C. and Clarkson, B.H. (1969) Walking patterns in healthy old men. *Journal of Gerontology*, **24**, 169–78.

Newell, K.M. (1991) Motor skill acquisition. *Annual Review of Psychology*, **42**, 213–317.

Norris, A.H., Lundy, T. and Shock, N.W. (1963). Trends in selected indices of body composition in men between the ages 30 and 80 years. *Annals NY Academy of Sciences*, 623–39.

O'Connell, A.L. and Gardiner, E.B. (1972) *Understanding the scientific basis of human movement*, Williams and Wilkins, Baltimore.

Oetel, G. (1986) Changes in human skeletal muscles due to ageing. *Acta Neuropathologica*, **69**, 309–13.

Øster, J. (1953) *Mongolism*, Danish Science Press, Copenhagen.

Paine, R.S. and Oppe, T. (1966) *The neurological examination of children*, Clinics of Developmental Medicine No. 20/21, Spastics International Medical Publications, London.

Paine, R.S., Donovan, D.E., Brazelton, T.B., Droorbaugh, J.E., Hubbell, J.P. and Sears, E.M. (1964) The evolution of postural reflexes in normal infants and in the presence of chronic brain syndromes, *Neurology*, 1 (14), 1036–48.

Palisano, R.J. (1988) Motor development, in *Human Development for Occupational and Physical Therapists*, (ed. M.A. Short-De Graff), Williams and Wilkins, Baltimore, pp. 445–77.

Parker, A. W. and James, B. (1985). Age changes in the flexibility of Down's syndrome children. *Journal of Mental Deficiency Research*, 29 (3), 207–18.

Parker, A.W., Bronks, R., and Snyder, C.W. (1986) Walking patterns in Down's syndrome, *Journal of Mental Deficiency Research*, 30 (4), 317–30.

Parker, A.W. and Bronks, R. (1980) Gait of children with Down syndrome, *Archives of Physical Medicine Rehabilitation*, 61, 345–51.

Patterson, D. (1987) The causes of Down syndrome, *Scientific American*, 257, 42–8.

Payne, V.G. and Isaacs, L.D. (1991) *Human Motor Development: A Lifespan Approach*, Mayfield Publishing Co., California.

Peiper, A. (1963) *Cerebral Function in Infancy and Childhood*, The International Behavioural Science Series, Translation of 3rd edition by B. and H. Naglar, Pub. Consultants Bureau, New York.

Pieterse, M., Bochner, S. and Bettison, S. (eds) (1988) *Early intervention for children with disabilities: the Australian experience*, Special Education Centre, Macquarie University, Sydney.

Pieterse, M. and Treloar, R. (1981) *The Down's syndrome program*, Progress Report, Macquarie University, Sydney.

Pitetti, K.H., Fernandez, J.E., Pizarro, D.C. and Stubbs, N.B. (1988) Field Testing: Assessing the physical fitness of mildly mentally retarded individuals. *Adapted Physical Activity Quarterly*, 5, 318–31.

Pizarro, D.C. (1990) Reliability of the health-related fitness test for mainstreamed educable and trainable mentally handicapped adolescents. *Adapted Physical Activity Quarterly*, 7, 240–48.

Prechtl, H.F.R. (1977) *The Neurological Examination of the Full-term Newborn Infant*, 2nd edn, Clinics of Developmental Medicine, No. 63, Spastics International Medical Publications, London.

Pueschel, S.M. (1987) Health concerns in persons with Down syndrome, in *New Perspectives on Down Syndrome*, (eds S.M. Pueschel, C. Tingey, J. Rynders, A.C. Crocker and D.M. Crutcher), Paul H. Brookes, Baltimore, pp. 113–33.

Pueschel, S.M. (1988) The biology of the maturing person with Down syndrome, in *The Young Person with Down Syndrome: Transition from Adolescence to Adulthood*, (ed. S.M. Pueschel), Paul H. Brookes, Baltimore, pp. 23–34.

Pueschel, S.M. and Pezzullo, J.C. (1985) Thyroid dysfunction in

Downs Syndrome, *American Journal of Diseases of Children*, **139**, 636–9.

Putnam, J.W., Pueschel, S.M. and Gorder-Holman, J. (1988) Community participation of youths and adults with Down syndrome, in *The Young Person with Down Syndrome: Transition from Adolescence to Adulthood*, (ed. S. M. Pueschel), Paul H. Brookes, Baltimore, pp. 77–92.

Raab, D.M., Agre, J.C., McAdam, M. and Smith, E.L. (1988) Light resistance and stretching exercise in elderly women: effect upon flexibility. *Archives of Physical Medicine and Rehabilitation*, **69**, 268–72.

Rankine-Wilson, J. (1980) *Prophylactic effects of exercise programs for the elderly*, paper presented at the Human Adaptation Conference, Cumberland College of Health Sciences, Sydney.

Rarick, G.L. and Seefeldt, V. (1974) Observations from longitudinal data on growth in stature and sitting height of children with Down's syndrome. *Journal of Mental Deficiency*, **18**, 63–78.

Rast, M.M. and Harris, S.R. (1985) Motor control in infants with Down syndrome, *Developmental Medicine and Child Neurology*, **27** (5), 682–5.

Reed, E.S. (1989) Changing theories of postural development, in *Development of Posture and Gait across the Life Span*, (eds. M.H. Woollacott and A. Shumway-Cook), University of South Carolina, Columbia, S.C., pp. 3–24.

Reed, R.B., Pueschel, S.M., Schnell, R.R. and Cronk, C.E. (1980) Interrelationships of biological environmental, and competency variables in young children with Down's syndrome, *Applied Research in Mental Retardation*, **1** (3–4), 161–74.

Reid, G. (1987) Physical Activity Programming, in *Current Approaches to Down's Syndrome*, (eds D. Lane and B. Stratford), Cassell, Gillingham, Kent, pp. 219–41.

Riguet, C.B. and Taylor, N.D. (1981) Symbolic play in autistic Down's and normal children of equivalent mental age. *Journal of Autism and Developmental Disorders*, **11**, 439–48.

Robinson, R.J. (1966) Assessment of gestational age by neurological examination. *Archives of Diseases of Children*, **41**, 437–47.

Rogers, J.C. (1987) Selection of evaluation instruments, in *A Therapist's Guide to Pediatric Assessment*, (eds L. King-Thomas and B.J. Hacker), Little, Brown and Co., Boston, pp. 19–33.

Rokosz, F.M. (1987) The paradoxes of play. *Physical Educator*, **45** (1), 5–13.

Ropper, A.H. and Williams, R.S. (1980) Relationship between plaques, tangles, and dementia in Down syndrome. *Neurology*, **30**, 639–44.

Rosenbaum, D.A. (1991). *Human Motor Control*, Academic Press, San Diego.

Rosenbloom, L. and Horton, M.E. (1971) The maturation of fine prehension in young children. *Developmental Medicine and Child Neurology*, **13**, 3–8.

Rudelli, R.D. (1985) The syndrome of musculoskeletal aging, in *Aging and Developmental Disabilities*, (eds M.P. Janecki and H.M. Wisniewski), Paul H. Brookes, Baltimore, pp. 229–56.

Ryan, T.M. (1977) A comparison of selected basic gross motor skills of moderately retarded and normal children of middle childhood age utilizing the Ohio State University scale of intra gross motor assessment. *Dissertion Abstracts International 38, 2650A*.

Sailor, S., Goetz, L., Anderson, J., Hunt, P. and Gee, K. (1988) Research on community intensive instruction as a model for building functional, generalized skills, in *Generalization and Maintenance*, (eds R.H. Horner, G. Dunlap and R.L. Koegel), Paul H. Brookes, Baltimore, pp.67–98.

Sato, T., Akatsuka, H., Kito, K. and Tokoro, Y. (1984) Age changes in size and number of muscle fibers in human minor pectoral muscle. *Mechanisms of Ageing and Development*, **28**, 99–109.

Sato, T., Akatsuka, H., Kito, K., Tokoro, Y., Tauchi, H. and Kato, K. (1986) Age changes of myofibrils in human minor pectoral muscle. *Mechanisms of Ageing and Development*, **34**, 297–304.

Saunders, P. (1984), *Micros for handicapped users*, Helena Press, Whitby (North Yorks).

Savolainen, J., Komulainen, J., Vihko, V., Vaananen, K., Puranen, J. and Takala, T.E.S. (1988) Collagen synthesis and proteloytic activities in rat skeletal muscles: Effect of cast-immobilization in the lengthened and shortened positions. *Archives of Physical Medicine and Rehabilitation*, **69**, 964–9.

Scanlan, T.K. and Passer, M. (1981) Competitive stress and the youth sport experience. *Physical Educator*, **38** (3), 144–51.

Scelsi, R., Marchetti, C. and Poggi, P. (1980) Histochemical and ultrastructural aspects of m. vastus lateralis in sedentary old people (age 65–89 years). *Acta Neuropathologica*, **51**, 99–105.

Schapiro, M.B. and Rapoport, S.I. (1989) Basal metabolic rate in healthy Down's syndrome adults. *Journal of Mental Deficiency Research*, **33** (3), 211–19.

Schiemer, A. and Abroms, I. (1980) *The practical management of the developmentally disabled child*, Mosby, St Louis.

Schleien S.J., Kiernan, J. and Wehman, P. (1981) Evaluation of an age-appropriate leisure skills program for moderately retarded adults. *Education and Training of the Mentally Retarded*, **16**, 13–19.

Schloss, P.J., Smith, M.A. and Kiehl, W. (1986) Rec Club: A community centered approach to recreational development for adults with mild to moderate retardation. *Education and Training of the Mentally Retarded*, **21**, 282–8.

Schmidt, R.A. (1988) *Motor control and learning: A behavioral emphasis*, 2nd edn, Human Kinetics, Illinois.

Schneck, C.M. and Henderson, A. (1990) Descriptive analysis of the developmental progression of grip position for pencil and crayon control in nondysfunctional children. *American Journal of Occupational Therapy*, **44**, 893–900.

Schweber, M. (1987) Interrelation of Alzheimer disease and Down syndrome, in *New perspectives on Down syndrome*, (eds. S.M. Pueschel, C. Tingey, J. Rynders, A.C. Crocker, and D.M. Crutcher), Paul H. Brookes, Baltimore, pp. 135–44.

Schwethelm, B., and Mahoney, G. (1986) Task persistence among organically impaired mentally retarded children. *American Journal of Mental Deficiency*, **90** (4), 432–9.

Seagoe, M.V. (1964) *Yesterday was Tuesday, all day and all night: The story of a unique education*, Little Brown, Toronto.

Seefeldt, V. and Haubenstricker, J. (1982) Patterns, Phases or Stages: An analytical model for study of developmental movement, in *The Development of Movement Control and Co-ordination*, (eds J.A.S. Kelso and J.E. Clark), John Wiley and Sons, pp. 309–18.

Seidl, C., Reid, G. and Montgomery, D.L. (1987) A critique of cardiovascular fitness testing with mentally retarded persons. *Adapted Physical Activity Quarterly*, **4**, 106–16.

Selikowitz, M.(1990) *Down syndrome: The Facts*, Oxford University Press, Oxford.

Seltzer, G.B. (1985) Selected psychological processes and aging among older developmentally disabled persons, in *Aging and Developmental Disabilities*, (eds M.P. Janecki and H.M. Wisniewski), Paul H. Brookes, Baltimore, pp. 211–323.

Share, J.B. and French, R.W. (1974) Early motor development in Down's syndrome children. *Mental Retardation*, **12** (6), 23.

Shepherd, R. (1979) Problem analysis with Down's syndrome infants. *Australian Journal of Physiotherapy: Pediatric Monograph*, 117–24.

Sherborne, V. (1982) Movement and the Mentally Disabled, in *Proceedings of the VII Commonwealth and International Conference on Sport, Physical Education, Recreation and Dance*, (eds M.L. Howell and K. Vassella), **5**, 33–6.

Sherborne, V. (1990) *Development and Movement for Children*, Cambridge University Press, Cambridge.

Sheridan, M. (1977) *Spontaneous Play in Early Childhood from Birth to Six Years*, NFER Publishing Company.

Sherrill, C. (ed.) (1988) *Leadership Training in Adapted Physical Education*, Human Kinetics, Champaign, Illinois.

Shock, N.W. and Norris, A.H. (1970) Neuromuscular co-ordination as a factor in age changes in muscular exercise, in *Medicine and Sport*, Vol 4, (eds D. Brunner and E. Jokl), University Park Press, Baltimore, pp. 92–9.

Shumway-Cook, A. and Woollacott, M.H. (1985) Dynamics of postural control in the child with Down syndrome. *Physical Therapy*, **65** (9), 1315–22.

Sidney, K.H., Shephard, R.J. and Harrison, J.E. (1977) Endurance training and body composition of the elderly. *American Journal Clinical Nutrition*, **30**, 326–33.

Sidney, K.H. and Shephard, R.J. (1978) Frequency and intensity of exercise training for elderly subjects. *Medicine and Science in Sports*, **10**, 125–31.

Silk, G. (1989) Creative movement for people who are developmentally disabled. *JOPERD*, **60** (9), 56–8.

Sim, L.J. and Stewart, C. (1984) The effects of videotape feedback on the standing broad jump performances of mildly and moderately mentally retarded adults. *Physical Educator*, **41** (1), 21–9.

Skerlj, B. (1959) Age changes in fat distribution in the female body. *Acta Anatomica*, **38**, 56–63.

Skerjl, B., Brozek, J. and Hunt, E.E. (1953). Body build in women. *American Journal of Physical Anthropology*, **11**, 577–99.

Skinner, H.B., Barrack, R.L. and Cook, S.D. (1984) Age-related decline in proprioception. *Clinical Orthopaedics*, **184**, 208–11.

Sloper, P., Glenn, S.M. and Cunningham, C.C. (1986) The effects of intensity of training on sensori-motor development in infants with Down syndrome. *Journal of Mental Deficiency Research*, **30**, 149–62.

Sloper, P., Turner, S., Knussen, C., and Cunningham, C. (1990) Social life of school children with Down syndrome. *Child: Care, Health and Development*, **16**, 235–51.

Smith, J.R. and Walker, J.M. (1983) Knee and elbow range of motion in healthy older individuals. *Physical and Occupational Therapy in Geriatrics*, **2** (4), 31–8.

Smyth, M.M. (1984) Perception and action, in *The Psychology of Human Movement*, (eds M.M. Smyth and M. Wing), Academic Press, London, pp. 119–52.

Smyth, M.M. and Wing, A.M. (eds) (1984). *The Psychology of Human Movement*, Academic Press, London.

Sokoloff, L. (1969) *The biology of degenerative joint disease*, University of Chicago Press, Chicago.

Sorce, J.F. and Emde, R.N. (1982) The meaning of infant emotional expressions: Regularities in caregiving responses in normal and Down's syndrome infants. *Journal of Child Psychology and Psychiatry*, **23** (2), 145–58.

Sovik, N. and Arnsten, O. (1991) A developmental study of the relationship between movement patterns in letter combinations and writing, in *Development of Graphic Skills*, (eds J. Wann, A.M. Wing and N. Sovik), Academic Press, London, pp. 77–89.

Stahlberg, E. and Fawcett, P.R.W. (1982) Macro EMG in healthy subjects of different ages. *Journal of Neurology, Neurosurgery and Psychiatry*, **45**, 870–78.

Stewart, D. (1990) *The Right to Movement: Motor Development in Every School*, Falmer Press, London.

Stipek, D. and MacIver, D. (1989) Developmental change in children's assessment of intellectual competence. *Child Development*, **60** (3), 521–38.

Stockmeyer, S.A. (1980) A sensori-motor approach to treatment, in *Physical Therapy Services in the Developmental Disabilities*, (eds P.H. Pearson and C.E. Williams, Charles C. Thomas, Springfield, Illinois, pp. 186–22.

Stoudt, H.W. (1981) The anthropometry of the elderly. *Human Factors*, **23**, 29–37.

Stratford, B. (1987) Learning and knowing: The education of Down's syndrome children, in *Current Approaches to Down's Syndrome*, (eds D. Lane and B. Stratford), Cassell, Gillingham, Kent, pp. 149–66.

Stratford, B. (1989) *Down syndrome: Past, present and future*, Penguin, London.

Stratford, B. and Ching, E.Y. (1989) Responses to music and movement in the development of children with Down's syndrome. *Journal of Mental Deficiency Research*, **33**, 13–24.

Stratford, B. and Steele, J. (1985) Incidence and prevalence of Down's syndrome: a discussion and report. *Journal of Mental Deficiency Research*, **29** (1), 95–107.

Sugden, D.A. and Keogh, J.F. (1990) *Problems in Movement Skill Development*, University of South Carolina, Columbia, S.C.

Suominen, H., Heikkinen, E., Liesen, H. and Hollman, W. (1977) Effects of 8 weeks endurance training on skeletal muscle metabolism in 66–70-year old sedentary men. *European Journal of Applied Physiology*, **37**, 173–80.

Thase, M.E. (1982a) Longevity and mortality in Down's syndrome. *Journal of Mental Deficiency Research*, **26**, 177–92.

Thase, M.E. (1982b) Reversible dementia in Down's syndrome. *Journal of Mental Deficiency Research*, **26**, 111–13.

Thase, M.E. (1988) The relationship between Down syndrome and Alzheimer's disease, in *The Psychobiology of Down Syndrome*, (ed. L. Nadel), MIT Press, Cambridge, Mass., pp. 345–68.

Thelen, E. (1989) The (re)discovery of motor development: learning new things from an old field. *Developmental Psychology*, **25** (6), 946–9.

Thelen, E. and Ulrich, B.D. (1991) Hidden skills. *Monographs of the Society for Research in Child Development*, **56** (1), 1–98.

Titus, J.A. and Watkinson, E.J. (1987) Effects of segregated and integrated programs on participation and social interaction of moderately mentally handicapped children in play. *Adapted Physical Activity Quarterly*, **4**, 204–19.

Touwen, B.C.L. (1971) A study on the development of some motor phenomena in infancy. *Developmental Medicine and Child Neurology*, **13**, 435–46.

Touwen, B.C.L. (1976) *Neurological development in infancy*, Clinics of Developmental Medicine Pub. Spastics International Medical Publications, London.

Tredwell, S.J., Newman, D.E. and Lockitch, G. (1990) Instability of the upper cervical spine in Down syndrome. *Journal of Pediatric Orthopedics*, **10** (5), 602–6.

Twitchell, T.W. (1954) Sensory factors in purposive movement. *Journal of Neurophysiology*, **17**, 239–42.

Twomey, L. (1981) Age related changes in the structure and dynamics of the lumbar spine, in *Human Adaptation*, (eds P. Russo and G. Gass), Cumberland College of Health Sciences, Sydney, pp. 281–93.

Tzankoff, S.P. and Norris, A.H. (1977) Effect of muscle mass decrease on age-related BMR changes. *Journal of Applied Physiology*, **43**, 12–16.

Tzankoff, S.P., Robinson, S., Pyke, F.S. and Brawn, C.A. (1972) Physiological adjustment to work in older men as affected by physical training. *Journal of Applied Physiology*, **33**, 346–50.

Umphred, D.A. and McCormack, G.L. (1990) Classification of common facilitatory and inhibitory treatment techniques, in *Neurological Rehabilitation*, 2nd edn, (ed. D.A. Umphred), C.V. Mosby, St Louis, pp. 72–117.

Vacc, N.N. and Vacc, N.A. (1979) Teaching manuscript writing to mentally retarded children. *Education and Training of the Mentally Retarded*, **14**, 286–91.

Vallerand, R.J. and Reid, G. (1990). Motivation and special populations: Theory, research, and implications regarding motor behavior, in *Problems in Movement Control*, (ed. G. Reid), Elsevier Science, Amsterdam, pp. 159–97.

Varnhagen, C.K., Das, J.P. and Varnhagen, S. (1987) Auditory and visual memory span: cognitive processing by TMR individuals with Down syndrome or other etiologies. *American Journal of Mental Deficiency*, **91**, 398–405.

Veietze, P.M., McCarthy, M., McQuiston, S., MacTurk, R. and Yarrow, L.J. (1983) Attention and exploratory behavior in infants with Down's syndrome, in *Infants Born at Risk: Physiological, Perceptual, and Cognitive Processes*, (eds T. Field and A. Sostek), Grune and Stratton, New York, pp. 251–70.

Wade, M.G. (1973) Biorhythms and activity of institutionalized mentally retarded persons diagnosed hyperactive. *American Journal of Mental Deficiency*, **78**, 262–7.

Walker, J.M. (1975) Generalized joint laxity in Igloolik Eskimos. *Human Biology*, **47**, 263–75.

Walker, J.M., Sue, D., Miles-Elkousy, N., Ford, G. and Trevelyan, H. (1984) Active mobility of the extremities in older subjects. *Physical Therapy*, **64**, 919–23.

Walker, P.S. (1977) *Human joints and their artificial replacements*, C.C. Thomas, Illinois.

Weinberg, R.S. (1981) Why kids play or do not play organised sports. *Physical Educator*, May, pp. 71–6.

Whiteman, B.C., Simpson, G. and Compton, W.C. (1986) Relationship of otitis media and language impairment in adolescents with Down syndrome. *Mental Retardation*, **24** (6), 353–6.

Wickstrom, R.L. (1983) *Fundamental Motor Patterns*, Lea and Febiger, Philadelphia.

Williams, P.E. and Goldspink, G. (1973) The effect of immobilization on the longitudinal growth of striated muscle fibres. *Journal of Anatomy*, **116**, 45–55.

Williams, P.E. and Goldspink, G. (1984) Connective tissue changes in immobilised muscle. *Journal of Anatomy*, **138**, 343–50.

Williamson, D.C. (1988) The transition swimming approach in

instructing people with disabilities, *British Journal of Physical Education*, **19**, 4–5, 159–162.

Wishart, J.G. (1991) Taking the initiative in learning: A developmental investigation of infants with Down syndrome. *International Journal of Disability, Development and Education*, **38** (1), 27–44.

Wisniewski, K.E., Miezejeski, C.M. and Hill, A.L. (1988) Neurological and psychological status of individuals with Down syndrome, in *The Psychobiology of Down Syndrome*, (ed. L. Nadel), MIT Press, Cambridge, Mass., pp. 315–43.

Woollacott, M.H. (1986) Gait and postural control in the aging adult, in *Disorders of posture and gait*, (eds W. Bles, W. and T. Brandt), Elsevier, Amsterdam, pp. 325–36.

Wyke, B. (1975) The neurological basis of movement: A developmental review, in *Movement and Child Development*, (ed. K. Holt), Clinics in Developmental Medicine No. 55, Pub. Spastics International Medical Publications, London, pp. 19–29.

Ziviani, J. and Elkins, J. (1984) An evaluation of handwriting performance, *Educational Review*, **36**, 249–61.

Ziviani, J. (1984) Some elaborations on handwriting speed in 7 to 14 years olds. *Perceptual and Motor Skills*, **58**, 535–9.

Author index

Subject index